Bulletproof
Confidence
and a
Kickass Body
through
Martial Arts Principles
and Training

MICHELLE HEXT

MichelleHext.com

BulletproofConfidenceKickassBody.com

DEDICATION

Delivering this book was part growing pains and part giving birth; there were tears, there were fears and there were breakthroughs of epic proportions.

To say this was an emotional experience would be an understatement; luckily I had amazing people in my life supporting me and keeping me sane and it is to these people I dedicate this book.

To my children Cody and Chloe – thank you for your patience and wisdom beyond your years.

To Tania, Lisa and Wendy – thanks for the laughs when I needed them, for the shoulders when I needed those, for your unwavering faith in me and your love. I think it's high time we had some bubbles.

CONTENTS

ACKNOWLEDGMENTS i

INTRODUCTION 1

PART ONE: 5

MY STORY – THE GOOD, THE BAD, AND THE UGLY

PART TWO: 49

BULLETPROOF CONFIDENCE

PART THREE: 91

TRAINING YOUR WAY TO A KICKASS BODY

ABOUT THE AUTHOR 122

ACKNOWLEDGMENTS

Wow! Where do I start…..?

The challenge here is to keep this part shorter than the book itself, because I have many, many people who have helped me bring this book to fruition:

Cody and Chloe: I got lucky, very lucky, as a mum. I have been gifted two amazing souls. Like all kids they are charged with the task of trying to drive their mother insane with worry, but they are also kind, insightful, loving, independent and funny. My greatest pleasure is seeing how much they love and care for each other and anyone who messes with their sibling had better look out! I love you guys, you make me a better person.

Mum: No doubt about it, mum and I have had our ups and downs. We are very alike in many ways – we share the same sense of humour, the same pragmatic approach to things and both have a very acute BS meter.

Mum, I love you, I know you did the best you could and I know there were many, many good times along the way. Here's to moving on and spending some more time together.

My family: My aunties, uncles, brothers and sister, and everyone in between. We are a whacky lot but I wouldn't trade you for the world. See you at Christmas xx

My girls: My girls… my amazing students at PUSH, my Rip It UP Challenge Ladies, my Glow ladies, my Facebook ladies, my girlfriends. You guys are my inspiration, every single one of you. Without you I would have still been looking to find my place in the world. You helped me to see what I do best, celebrated every success I have had along the way and also picked me up when things got tough. You light up my life and make every day a blessing. I would not be a man for quids. Cam, despite not being a girl, you rate just as highly ☺

My instructors: Mr Chang. Mr Chang is no longer with us, but his influence on my life lingers and I am truly grateful for having been able to spend time with such a wonderful man. Mr Chang walked me down the aisle (the first time!!) and was the first person to visit Cody when he was born. He also gifted Cody his middle name 'Tae Soo', which means to grow big, stand strong and have a long life. **Greg.** Knowing you changed my world. I feel very blessed to have been your student and will always consider myself so. Things between us were rough for far too long and I'm so glad we have finally found peace with each other and can now remember the good times. It is also truly wonderful to finally be able to parent our amazing kids together.

INTRODUCTION

Apparently everyone has a book in them… clearly me included.

I just wasn't sure what that book would be about, but I did know writing it would open a can of worms I wasn't sure I was ready for!

My life is defined by martial arts, fitness and a fierce mindset, so I knew it had to be a book about training and mindset. But my life has also been what you could describe as… well, let's just say I have had to be resilient and show great strength and determination to get through some of it.

I refused to write a book wrapping up the same old stuff with the addition of some secret recipe, ratio or ingredient that would help to sell a book.

I refused to jump on the bandwagon of selling crap for dollars.

I refused to write something I would not pay good money for.

I wanted to write a book that meant something and that would challenge the reader and hopefully change their life in some way.

Much like I helped to changed Mrunal's life. She shares her story below:

"I remember when I first approached you for help. I was frustrated because I was feeling sick all the time and my lack of energy and enthusiasm were causing a few problems. The moment I read your profile on the Push Taekwondo website and went through all the testimonials, I knew I had to meet you. And it is definitely one of the best decisions I've ever taken in my life.

When I first saw you, I could see the passion that comes from strong conviction, I could see the empathy and understanding in your eyes, but above all, I could sense a strong, free spirit. I knew then that taking personal training with you would be a start of something special that I would treasure all my life.

Whenever I suffered from lack of confidence (which was frequent back then as I couldn't even do five push-ups on my knees), you'd always remind me that we all have to start somewhere. It became easier to keep my goals in mind. I gained a better understanding of nutrition and reading labels. When I came to see you for the first time, I had just been through months of a no-carb diet which had completely ruined my metabolism. You guided me in my nutrition and forced me to eat everything again but in the right portions, at the right time and in the right way. And as you said time and again, eating more will help me reduce weight, not dieting. And you were so correct.

You supported me to take up Taekwondo when I completed my personal training. And again, I've never once regretted that decision. I can safely say I have discovered another passion in my life in Taekwondo. I always lacked discipline and patience in my life and learning this martial art has given me the tools to control myself.

Learning this Martial Art has brought a discipline into my life; something I have always strived to achieve but failed. I absolutely love your way of teaching. When you perform, it inspires all of the class to do better. I have seen a few different teachers now, but many only teach Taekwondo to award belts; they exude no passion. You teach to not only create a fierce and competitive athletes, but also to change the lives of women through empowerment and positivity.

Push is one of a kind. Every time I step into the dojang, I feel at peace. I look forward to the class. Because of the values you espouse at Push, there is a unique camaraderie between all the girls and women, as we all have mutual respect and are willing to help each other. Yet, when we spar, we become competitors. It is an eclectic mix of personalities. And I cannot imagine having better females to learn, spar and grow with. YOU have created this.

I want to take this opportunity to Thank You for all that you have done for me. You teach, inspire and sometimes push (just kidding!) me to become better. I wish you all the very best for everything that

you take on in your life. Your strength is a force to be reckoned with. And I feel proud to call you my teacher.

Thank you Michelle

Mrunal"

What I promise about this book, is that what you read is deep from the heart and was written the same way I live my life – at full throttle!

I have been faced with some of life's tougher challenges and I know from speaking to 1000s of women over the years that my story is a powerful one that has resonated with many women, and I knew it just had to be told.

My Facebook friends agreed (and I hold them in VERY high regard!) and so the first section of this book is about my life and how I came to be where I am now; which is in the best shape of my life (mentally and physically) at the age of 44, doing what I love most in the world working with amazing women every day, living with purpose and passion and living comfortably.

So without apology I am going to ask you to put on *your* big girl pants and come with me on the journey of my life story, in the hope of inspiring you to see that no matter where you are in life, you can chose to fight the good fight and come out on top.

You will notice that I use humour when I discuss some of my darkest moments and this is part of who I am – I don't take myself too seriously. I take what I do, and the impact I have on others, seriously, but I also like to laugh at myself and remember that life is how you choose to see it and how you choose to live it.

I'm not all about "woe is me" and I'm not assuming that you are broken, and need fixing; however anyone struggling with their weight or self-esteem usually has at least one thing holding them back, so you are not alone there.

I have needed, and still need, regular maintenance (on my mind and body) just as my car does and just as you do, just like we all do, so consider this book and what comes from it to be your "tune up".

I know a lot about challenges because life has thrown a few at me over the past 44 years (some of my own doing) and I know that without Martial Arts and fitness in my life things would be very different to how they are today.

I am often asked what my greatest strength is?

I believe I have several strengths, but I have to say that without a doubt, number one is my resilience and indomitable spirit.

My ability to bounce back from adversity and grow stronger and wiser for the experience.

The faith I have in myself that I cannot be broken.

That I can go toe to toe with any adversity that comes my way in this lifetime and know I will come out on top.

I'm like this in training too.

When it starts to hurt, when it gets hard, that is when I really switch on and start to enjoy the ride. Because here is where I know I am fitter, faster, stronger and tougher than most people. I am reminded that I can take more physical punishment than most people. I won't be broken. I take great pride and satisfaction in this, it reinforces all of the good things I know about myself.

In training is where I am at one with my indomitable spirit; training at intensity and getting through a tough training session reinforces that wherever I put my mind I can get my body to follow.

In the following pages I hope to take you on a life-changing journey that not only leaves you empowered, but also equipped with a set of life skills to enable you to develop the sort of bulletproof confidence you need to truly live the life you deserve and do it in a body you love living in… a kickass one!

For further information visit my websites at **MichelleHext.com** and **BulletproofConfidenceKickassBody.com**

PART ONE:

MY STORY –
THE GOOD, THE BAD, AND THE UGLY
(only not in any particular order!)

All of my life I have been a fighter in one way or another, and my fighting spirit has never let me down, it has in fact helped shape the person I am today.

And so let me share with you the abridged version of my life so far...

You can hear people tell you the same things a million times over, yet when you finally see them for yourself it's like you are hearing it for the very first time.

A sudden rush of images flows through my mind, much like a silent movie, fragments from my sometimes sad, sometimes incredible life.

At times the movie is fast, but it slows down enough at regular intervals for me to endure the pain of a memory with heart-wrenching clarity.

For years I'd been able to tell the story of my life as if it belonged to someone else because I had distanced myself from it for so long and was so used to shutting out the horror of it, that I felt no emotion.

Ripping the Band-Aid off my past and creating a big mess was painful, but as a result it helped me to finally experience real peace and healing, not the forced kind I was used to.

People who have heard my story are in awe at what I have been able to achieve given my start in life. I dismiss this with the immediate thought that I should be so much more, so much better, so much further along than I am now. What you see is nothing... I'm not finished, I'm not there yet; just wait until you can see what I really know I can do.

Before I continue, let me just remind you that I'm in a really good place now. I have two beautiful children, a business I am passionate about and that fulfils me and good friends. And while I imagine I'll always want to have more, do more and be more in my life, I now understand that this is what makes me me, and helps me to continually grow. It's also what got me to where I am now. I've discovered that for me contentment is only a fleeting thing so I know I need to enjoy it while it lasts!

LET'S START WITH THE GOOD...

MY NANA and PA...

My family (the one I grew up with) is broken and scattered, and even though it has been this way for many, many years now, at times it still bothers me.

I'm pretty sure this is because of my grandparents (Mum's parents) and the example they set for me. And I also imagine that my grandparents had a good few years with me before I came to acknowledge the constant presence of fear and anxiety in my life.

My Mum is one of five sisters – what a handful for my poor old Pa! Those girls were so full of mischief! And the stories they told were hilarious!

My sister and I could not get enough of their stories of the 'olden days'. I loved the way they laughed so much they would roll around laughing about the stuff they got up to – I wanted mine to be that life.

I wanted fun and laughter and love and camaraderie and ease.

I loved that they lived in the same house for their whole lives (I lost count of the number of homes we lived in by the time I left at 16, but it was up around the high 20s for sure), and their house was rowdy and fun and naughty.

I loved my Nana and Pa more than anything else in the whole wide world. As a small child I would often go to bed crying myself to sleep at the thought that they would die and leave me. I just couldn't stand the thought and it tore me up.

This was years before I knew they were both sick and it turned out that neither would live long enough to see me in my 20s, as they both died in their 50s.

My sweet nana developed Type 1 diabetes in her 20s after a bad car accident, but she also had a bunch of other things go wrong as a result of the experimental medicine she allowed them to practice on her. Nana also had Coeliac disease, she had had her thyroid removed and I can remember that on at least one occasion she had open heart surgery.

She suffered a lot in her short time on the planet, but you would never know it.

We went to visit Nana and Pa pretty much every day, and every day I would ask Nana, "How are you today Nan?" and every single time she would say, "Good Chell".

She obviously wasn't 'good' at all but she never, ever let on and always had a smile and was just so, so lovely.

My Pa was awesome!

Whilst I didn't know it then, I appreciate now that he was obviously a man before his time.

He practiced yoga and I can remember a photo of him doing a push-up off a chair with his body hovering horizontally – he was so strong!

He was also always making protein shakes and smoothies way before they became cool.

I can remember my mum telling me that as a child he used to make her a shake with eggs and milk and wheat germ because she refused to eat 'normal' food.

My Pa was a very popular man, he was a supervisor at the local Shire and everyone loved him.

Pa had his 'shed' down the back of the yard and I was instructed to whistle or sing as I was heading down the path. It was only many years later that I worked out it was to give the men fair warning I was on my way, so they wouldn't swear when I was around!

I can still remember vividly the surprised looks on the men's faces one particular time as I marched into the shed and proudly displayed the dollies

I had made from a packet of tampons. I had drawn faces on them and had them dangling off my fingers. I was running through the names of my tampon people and what they did for a living! Looking back this was priceless – the poor men were so indulgent, but I'm sure they wouldn't have known what had hit them!

I have some very fond memories of Pa and me sitting in his shed eating a flounder he had caught and cooked for me, solving the problems of the world.

One day he served up some sea snails and I ate every one of them because my pa had made them.

I know that if my Pa were alive today I could learn a lot from him about being fit and healthy.

My grandparents are sorely missed and I hope they knew how much I loved them, and just how much they helped shape my moral compass. Without even knowing, they taught me about unconditional love, kindness and compassion.

My Mum could hit me and yell at me as much as she wanted. My Dad could bellow, and hit, and be intimidating as much as he liked. But to no avail, I would rarely back down even as a small child. However, my Nana, on one single occasion, firmed up her softly-spoken voice and uttered one sentence. "Be good for your mother, you don't know what you are doing to her, I'm worried about her and you are not helping."

This from my Nana! The one person I could rely on to think of me as a good girl, no matter what. In my mind I thought that she didn't think that anymore, that I had ruined it!!! I will never forget the pain of that as long as I live. That said, I didn't blame her! In my opinion it was my *Mum's* fault for telling tales, and pretty much anyone and everyone else's fault for not understanding me!

NOTHING IS SIMPLE!

My Mum and Dad were boyfriend and girlfriend from the age of 13. My Dad was good to my Mum in the early days, and Mum obviously loved him, because after being told repeatedly they could not get married at 16 or 17, they decided in their wisdom that if Mum was pregnant they would *have* to get married! In 1968 my Mum unknowingly sacrificed all she could be, only to throw away many years of her life, living with a violent and very selfish man.

As is typical in our history, this isn't as simple as Mum getting pregnant and marrying Dad. Mum was still living at home and when she told her parents she was pregnant, Nana and Pa had a fit! She still wasn't allowed to get married and so Dad left the area looking for work. During that time Mum thought she had miscarried the baby, she told the news to her parents, only to then find out soon after that she was mistaken, Being young, immature and pregnant for the first time , I can only imagine she had some bleeding and jumped to the wrong conclusion. So instead of letting on she was in fact still pregnant, there she was, living at home in a bedroom shared with her four sisters, hiding her pregnancy.

Until she went into labour!

She hung on and on, thinking she could maybe wait till her parents went to work the next day, but as best laid plans often do, these ones went astray!

The whole house was woken up. I think my Auntie Karen had the job of waking Nana and Pa and breaking the happy news. Mum says she can still hear Pa yelling, "You live in the same house as your daughter and still don't know she's bloody pregnant. Well I'm not driving her to the hospital!"

Of course he did drive her to the hospital and a few days later I came home to a proud and adoring Pa and Nana and a hoard of fussing aunties.

I could write a whole book on my aunties and the fun we used to have.

I can remember lying in bed with my Auntie Jacqui as she wrote letters on my back and I had to guess them. She would do this for hours!

I spent a lot of time with my Auntie Karen and Uncle Dez as well.

My auntie Karen was a hairdresser and had a hair salon in the seaside town of Rye (on the Mornington Peninsula in Victoria) and I used to walk there after school.

She had set up a basin and hair dummy for me so I could 'play' hairdresser. I loved it.

My Uncle Dez was very significant in my life because, apart from my Pa, he was the only man I knew who loved me 100% and who I trusted not to hurt me.

My Uncle Dez and I used to sit upstairs for hours in their flat above the hair salon going through the Guinness Book of Records rolling around laughing at some of the stuff in there.

He taught me to be curious and be interested in many different things.

This stuff is 'good', this is the stuff I love to recall. It helps to balance out the bad.

AND NOW FOR SOME BAD
(WITH A FEW GOOD BITS)

When I was six months old, Pa finally let Mum and Dad get married and our little family moved into a flat not far from my grandparents. Also living in those flats was a group of young men all serving in the army. My Dad had always fancied himself as a tough guy. He had been a Golden Gloves Boxing Champion, as had his brothers and his father. He also enjoyed playing footy and cricket, and loved to drink with the boys.

It seems that something went very wrong for my Dad about now. From the time they got married, something in him changed. His personality switched and he began to routinely beat my mother. Mum says she can still remember the first time. She couldn't get over the shock of it. From then on he began to spend most nights out getting smashed with the boys, and then he'd come home and use Mum, and later us kids, as a punching bag … Hmmm… good guy, my Dad!

I don't know how old I was exactly, but I can remember asking enough questions to work out I was born 'out of wedlock'. I don't think I got over the indignation of this for a very long time. Ironic really when this was the least of my problems!

Fast forward now to several years later when my Mum became pregnant with my youngest brother. She wasn't yet married to my stepdad, and I had a fit! I was around 12 years old and I ran away from home. When I was finally ready to return, I insisted they get married, because I couldn't stand the humiliation of them having a baby born 'out of wedlock' just as I had been. And this was in 1982! However, many years later when I became pregnant with my first child, I also wasn't married and it horrified me! So much so that I insisted that my partner and I must get married immediately. For reasons that I will discuss in the following chapters, this marriage ended in divorce.

(My Mum and then-stepdad's marriage didn't last either.)

I married again, on the rebound, not long after my first divorce. This marriage lasted less than 12 months and I was out of there almost as quickly as I had gone into it.

My Mum and I were two all!

Sadly, I went on to get married a third time and although this relationship lasted a decade, it also eventually failed. Clearly I was a slow learner! I've been told I should "never say never" but there is a deep part of me that truly believes I don't have the right to ever get married again. This isn't me giving up on being in a committed loving relationship; however it just seems that marriage is the kiss of death for me and I'm not sure I am willing to take the risk again…

I once read about a man who had been abandoned by his mother as a baby. He had then lived in foster care and institutions all his life. The story was, in effect, saying that because he had never been loved, he never learned how to love. It hit me like a hammer! I had never been shown how to have a loving, equal relationship and unfortunately I paid for this (as did my partners) by way of failed marriage after failed marriage.

I just couldn't work out why I always ended up in relationships destined to fail. In the early days there was always yelling, screaming and someone leaving. At that time I remember thinking, "This is really crap, I don't need this, I hate this."

Eventually the realization dawned on me that this was what I thought relationships were all about. I was playing out my parents' marriage, again and again! Consequently my brother and sister both lived through failed marriages.

I want to make it clear, however, that I am not blaming anyone else for my failed marriages. My parents didn't set out to create this pattern of behaviour for me. But it does go to show that it is far more powerful to lead by example than it is to expect others to "Do what I say not what I do!"

Let me reiterate that you may hear this and understand it intellectually, but *until* you get it, it's like you haven't heard the concept before. Your brain says, "Oh, that's what all that was about and why people got so fired up about this stuff, because it's true – now I get it".

For a fairly smart girl, it took me a lot to 'get it'. The penny finally dropped when I thought to myself, "These guys are quite possibly all idiots but they didn't date each other. I'm the common denominator here, so what's up with me and why am I choosing them and this constant state of drama?"

The simple answer was that I'd never known any other way of life.

Whilst my memory is at times fuzzy on some of the time frames of my early childhood (especially given I tried so hard for many years to forget most of it!), I'm relying on the best memory I have; however some time frames may be inaccurate but my recall of the events along the way is crystal clear.

MY LIFE FELL APART

I was about six years old when my auntie's fiancé started molesting me.

My life had started falling apart and no-one noticed.

I remember the day I was sitting in church with Nana at my auntie's wedding. I was bawling my eyes out. I couldn't stop thinking about what my soon-to-be-uncle had done to me and now my auntie was about to marry him. I remember sitting there thinking that this was it and that it would never stop, as he was now here for good. Nana was smiling adoringly down at me, asking me what was wrong and trying to comfort me. All I could think to tell her was that I was sad knowing I'd miss my auntie not living with her and Pa anymore. There was just no way I could tell my beautiful Nana the truth.

I remember being so afraid to go to the toilet when we visited my auntie at her new house. 'He' would ALWAYS be waiting for me when I came out of the toilet. He'd take me into his (soon to be born) child's room, pull my pants down, and get into the single bed with me. He'd ask me what I was thinking. What was I thinking? I was thinking, "Why doesn't someone come looking for me?" "Why doesn't someone help me?" Yet at the same time I was hoping that no-one would discover this shameful thing. That's what I was thinking!!

My Mum and Dad were only three rooms away. I would beg my sister to come to the toilet with me, but she never would, and now many years later knowing what had happened, she still harbours guilt about this.

At one point I remember 'he' warned me that if I told anyone about the things he was doing to me, my auntie would lose the baby she was carrying.

Other times he would say that my Nana would die if she ever found out what I had done. So of course I didn't tell. But I did do everything I could to avoid staying at their place.

Late one night when I was about ten I had a girlfriend staying over. She was a few years older than me, and I took the opportunity to share some of the more gory details with her and ask her if anything like that had ever happened to her. She looked at me horrified and said, "NO! Did it happen to you?"

I said, "NO! I was just wondering?"

I eventually went to sleep mortified that this wasn't something that happened to all girls my age.

The next thing I knew I was woken by my Mum who had come racing into my bedroom, yelling and firing questions at me. I mistook this for anger and thought I was in big trouble, as I had been conditioned by 'him' to believe I would be.

My friend, Leanne, had waited until I was asleep and then she had gone and told Mum what I had told her.

I remember Mum's interrogation went something like this…

"Is 'X' touching you?"

"No."

"TELL ME!"

"He isn't!"

"Well, that's not what Leanne told me! Tell me what he's been doing to you!"

I was not only peeved at Leanne for being a dobber, I was also mortified and scared to death. Now as an adult looking back, I know I owe her such gratitude. Who knows how long the physical and mental abuse would have continued if she hadn't intervened and told Mum, because there was no way I was going to tell anyone.

Mum eventually calmed down enough to let me know I wasn't in trouble, but that I really needed to tell her everything. She also asked why I hadn't told her.

I told her it was because I believed what 'he' had told me – that if I did tell it would lead to Nana dying (who was my favourite person in the whole world and was already sick), to my auntie losing her baby – and the worry that no-one would believe me anyway. I was also scared my Dad would lose it and kill him for what he had done to me, given what a violent man he was.

All of these were paralysing fears and responsibilities for a then-ten-year-old to be burdened with because, despite the dysfunction within my family, they still meant everything to me and I still wanted them to love me.

Needless to say whilst the last four or so years of my life had been a living hell, the following weeks and months of my life as the truth came out were also extremely uncomfortable.

All I wanted to do was get on with my life. I didn't want to talk about it. I didn't want to think about it. I just wanted to forget the whole thing had happened and enjoy living without having to be constantly filled with fear, at least about that.

At this point the domestic violence I was exposed to as a child was still rife, but compared to the sexual abuse I had endured, it was a walk in the park.

My auntie eventually left my uncle and went to live in another State. Although the behaviour of her husband was to some extent responsible for her becoming a drug addict, I felt like a lot of it was my fault and as a result, I had to live with the guilt. It was many decades later before we could talk about everything that had happened, including the guilt that I carried thinking I was to blame for her marriage demise and addiction.

In my mind I believed that my telling about the abuse was what made her become an addict, and I still believed this to be a fact right up until my late 30s.

Sadly the conversation I needed to have with her for over two decades came just before she passed away from lung cancer just before her fiftieth birthday. It meant the world to me to hear from her that she didn't blame me for what her life had become, because I had carried that guilt with me for a very long time. That one conversation at her death bed gave both of us a lot of peace and closure. I just wish we had done it sooner.

'HE' turned up at my auntie's funeral (I know!) and it had been close to 30 years since I had last seen him. Let's just say I took the opportunity to let him know in no uncertain terms I was not his biggest fan, that he wasn't welcome and 'kicked him' out of the wake.

I was proud of the fact I didn't literally 'kick' his head off his shoulders, like I could (and should??) have done, but instead remained very calm and controlled and kept the upper hand. To watch him scurry away at lightning speed like the rat that he was gave me a lot of satisfaction.

But not for long...

For years I had dreamed about the day we would meet again, and how awesome I would feel confronting him as an adult. I believed that I would be healed, but I was very sadly mistaken.

I fell apart for a while after that encounter and everything that flowed from it. I found myself in a black hole for months.

For example, during those months, when my family left the house for the day, although I was dressed for the gym, I never went there. I would sit on the couch and watch television all day, every day. Depression (although I could never bring myself to call it that for fear of it actually being so) had set in.

At the time I was running an online business and I had become the inspiration for a lot of women to lose weight and change their lives. Never had I felt like such a hypocrite.

No-one ever knew what I was going through; I kept it to myself and worked through it, but at times I wondered if it would ever end.

I should be close to my cousin (the daughter of my auntie and that uncle), but I know nothing about who she is as a person. I could never get over the guilt of breaking up her family and blaming myself for her Mum turning into an addict. I never knew what she had been told about her father, and I just didn't ever want to be in a position where I would put my foot in it with her.

Many years later it emerged that a number of girls were raped near a sports oval close to where my uncle lived. I just knew it was 'him'. He eventually moved interstate so he could be close to his daughter, and for years this was a source of constant anxiety for me.

During this time one of my other aunties, who was aware of what had happened to me as a child, made a phone call to the local Police Department where he lived, informing them of his past. He subsequently disappeared for several years. I don't know for certain, but my aunties believe he ended up in jail and had a pretty hard time of it. Karma is a good thing!

I could now abandon my daydreams of picking him up in a bar somewhere (he wouldn't recognize me, of course) and seeking my revenge!!!

I don't remember how long after the truth about the abuse came out that Mum finally decided to leave Dad but in my mind it was maybe a year. By this time I was around 11 and had witnessed first-hand my dad kicking the crap out of Mum and calling her names that I still can't repeat. I had also personally borne the brunt of his anger; I still think my brother and sister were relatively unscathed (at least physically) at this point.

When I was young I used to think Mum was weak for staying with my Dad and I couldn't understand why she didn't just leave. Now that I understand more about domestic violence, I know how strong she was to stay and live with that day after day. I also understand the fear she had about leaving.

Mum and my future stepdad had begun spending time together and obviously had feelings for each other and it was he who gave her the strength to leave.

Not long after my mum and future stepdad got together, I remember my Dad telling us kids we were all going on a holiday to Queensland. I wasn't having a bar of it, I was staying with my Mum; however my brother and sister decided to go as Dad could be very convincing. I stayed with Mum and watched suspiciously as my soon-to-be stepfather courted my mother and at the same time he seemed to be befriending me. I wasn't playing ball for one second, I could smell a rat! For some reason despite everything, I was still loyal to my Dad even though I had been privy to his violence and abuse of our family.

I later found out that Dad had taken the kids without permission and Mum had had detectives trying to track him down in Queensland all that week. Dad was forced to bring my brother and sister back to my Mum, and for a while we all had a pretty good time – just my Mum and me, and my brother and sister, and this is how I wanted it to stay. I finally felt as though I had my Mum for real.

And then Dad found out about Mum's new boyfriend.

Mum and her boyfriend moved in together and so the next round began.

This was heralded by Dad pulling up in our driveway and screaming obscenities at Mum and her boyfriend for the entire neighbourhood to hear. This then gave way to my good old Dad breaking in the door, dragging my soon-to-be-stepdad down the back steps and giving him a hiding.

As kids this was terrifying; it always happened at night in the dark, which made it seem all the worse. I'm sure over time we couldn't help but listen out for my Dad's arrival.

My Dad would then storm into our house and grab my little brother, who was about four at the time, and start throwing open cupboards looking for my brother's things. He told us he was taking my brother with him and would we come too? I mean who wouldn't right???!! We cried and told him we loved him and would still visit him every day after school. I was scared of him and felt sorry for him at the same time.

He would leave; we would put things back together again, patch up my stepdad, pick up the broken stuff and cry for my brother and my Mum, who was completely distraught.

A few days later my brother would be unceremoniously dumped back home with complaints of him being a "f#@king little mummy's boy". My brother cried a lot because he missed Mum (and more than likely because of the way my Dad behaved during that time along with seeing what had gone on the previous night), and so Dad would torment him about his tears and my brother would cry his little heart out.

I am pretty sure my brother has never lived a peaceful day in his life and I would like to see my Dad pay for this, but he doesn't seem to have a conscience and so it will never happen. My brother has opened himself up to my Dad so many times and still does, even when he knows better and he is never surprised that Dad still does all he can to make him feel lower than a snake.

If I ever cried as an adult, it was over my brother – every time. He is a resilient little bugger, but living a life he should never ever have had to live. While I'm OK he is not, and I don't know whether he ever will be and this is a very tough thing to live with, because despite all that he has become, he is my baby brother.

Not far down the track we were shoved aside for Dad's new improved family. My brother copped an emotional hiding. My sister was ignored. However, I was the golden girl (which lead to a mountain load of guilt) and I was fed all the wonderful stories about how happy he was, so I could run along home and tell Mum and my stepdad all about it.

Back at Mum's I was running away (not too far) pretty often. I hated everyone. I couldn't cope with the fact that Mum and my stepdad were together and when I pulled the blankets back in a light-hearted moment one morning and saw them 'naked' that was my undoing.

A second similar occurrence, this time when we were staying at a caravan park, saw my stepdad chasing me around the caravan park at 2am in his jocks. I ran out of puff and figured I was safe to hide in the ladies' toilets because men weren't allowed in there. I was annoyed to find this wasn't foremost in my stepdad's mind as he dragged me kicking and screaming back to Mum, all the while trying to calm me down.

My stepdad still loves me today (even though I forget Father's day and his birthday) and he loved me then. I was a little spitfire and I made his life hell on earth, but bit by bit he broke my resolve to hate him forever. This resolve was being fed by my father of course.

My stepdad never ever hit me, not once, and while for most kids this would be a no-brainer this was a massive deal for me. He was always gentle and kind, but unfortunately he had far too many bad habits that my Mum just couldn't deal with. Given the last decade or so of her life I don't blame her, but the deterioration of their relationship was very sad to witness.

I don't think my stepdad ever really got over their break up, but for a long time now he and Mum have been fast friends and this is good for my heart. My stepdad had the best sense of humour! When we were kids he made us laugh until we couldn't breathe, and he was a big, gentle bear.

He certainly wasn't perfect, but he loved me and I loved him back and still do today.

I began to call my stepdad 'Dad' a long time after my brother and sister did. I think I saved 'the big day' for his birthday (always was dramatic) and he cried, and so did I, and we became firm friends ever after – faults and all (his and mine).

If I didn't know any better I would not have known from his behaviour that he wasn't my real dad; he loved me so much and I felt it very clearly.

Things were going pretty badly for me and Mum though. We were always fighting; at one point my stepdad had to break us apart when I lashed back at her. Mum constantly called me names, the worst one being a certain four letter word starting with 'C' – the one you just don't say! Especially to your child! She would lay into me with her hands or a wooden spoon or whatever was handy and one time was especially bad.

Reading my reader was always such a stressful time, because I always confused the words 'where' and 'were' and so I was anxious about those words before I even got to them. I stuffed them up every time and this lead to her frustration and me being hit; it was just rotten!

Another time my sister and I had to do the washing up and I KNEW it was my turn to wash (if you were born anytime around the 60s you no doubt recognise this particular argument!) and my sister said it was her turn to wash. Mum yelled at me to dry and I said, "Nu-uh, no way sister, not my turn" (if not those exact words then at least in that sentiment). It escalated as it often did, to the point where my Mum lost it and began whacking me and at one point I thought, "Ah-ha, I'll pretend to pass out!" Only to my surprise when I hit the deck she kept at it, so I got up and ran out and sat on the hill behind our caravan (yes, caravan!) until after dark, hating my life and hoping the dishes were done. I walked back in and Mum said, "Get the dishes done!" I seriously thought about firing up but was too sore and tired to argue, so I ended up giving her that one, much to my disgust!

WHERE IT ALL BEGAN

This was a weird time and it's hard to recall exact dates, but I know it was during Year 7.

We had been living in Dargo and then Rosedale for about two or three years, away from the crapola of Dad. In Grade 6 I was at Rosedale Primary School. I had made some friends and was all set to begin Year 7 at Sale High School. I had the uniform and everything!. Then the next thing you know – BANG – we are moving to Blairgowrie (hours away back on the Mornington Peninsula) and living in tents on a block of land and "HELLO you are going to Rosebud High School" – I nearly died! I remember living in those crappy tents – it rained a lot, we showered in the public showers on the Rye foreshore, and it wasn't at all enjoyable!

I was lucky enough to be able to contact a friend I had from Primary School and she met me at the front gate on the first day of High School. In the meantime my stepdad had raced out and bought me a uniform and school shoes. My uniform was too short and I was the only kid in school with black lace-up school shoes. My only saving grace was my friend had become a cool kid and no-one messed with her and by association no-one messed with me either!

My friend and I were very different and while I loved her, I couldn't get into the things she was into. Whilst we remained friends we didn't hang out for very long.

I never really fitted in at high school, but I can't say it scarred me for life. I know there were lots of tears and a lot of time spent feeling like a freak, but for the most part I just got on with it and spent a lot of time in the library; books became my salvation.

I wasn't prepared to put up with crap just to have friends and I'm still the same today! Give me a good book over a crappy friendship any day!

Fast forward a few years and let's just say home life and school life didn't get any better. I was told by my Mum that she was not spending money sending me back to school when I was wasting my time.

I left school at 14 and it was something that mortified me for years and years, because now on top of the stigma of having low income, domestic abuse, sexual abuse and divorced parents, I now had no education (in fact I put off writing this book and so many other things for so many years for fear it would show up my lack of formal education, something I had tried to hide).

I knew that if I was not to become a statistic I had a lot of work ahead of me.

Despite my circumstances I still had high hopes for myself. Funnily enough despite everything I think this came from my Mum.

I can remember her dreaming of the house she would have one day and I can remember she had a whole bunch of magazines and pages from magazines of the way she wanted her dream house to look.

I can remember finding a picture of a bedroom I loved, and Mum tore it out and promised I would have that room one day. While it didn't actually happen, I honestly believed at the time that it would!

Mum made me believe we would and could have anything we dreamed of. Winning TattsLotto featured heavily in our dream making. Now all these years later my Mum and her partner have in fact built more than one dream house. My Mum finally got to live out her dream and I am as pleased as anyone to see it.

Anyway, I digress (again!!)...

After I left school I had a cracking career in the Woolworths Deli – they tried me out on the register, but I just couldn't cut it – I don't know what the hell was going on there but being on the register freaked me out and I kept making stupid mistakes.

Over the years I had a few different jobs, mainly working in cafes, a shoe shop, that type of thing, and I wasted every cent I earned.

I moved out of home as soon as I could (I was about 16) and worked hard at being a grown up.

THE FIRST BOYFRIEND

When I was 16 I met my first 'real' boyfriend.

He was a few years older than me. I loved him but he annoyed the crap out of me A LOT and his Mum drove me up the wall. He didn't have the best start in life either but he had made good.

When I met him he was working on a farm for a very wealthy family and had very high hopes for himself. In the time we were together, he travelled and lived in the USA and UK and is now a captain for a major airline.

He taught me to strive for what I wanted and without him I'm not sure I would be where I am now, hard to say but maybe so.

Spending time with his wealthy employers and seeing other wealthy people through my hospitality job, my lack of education bothered me more and more.

I knew how to behave. I knew how to converse. I was proud of who I was becoming, but I felt dumb and ignorant having no education and not having travelled.

My boyfriend encouraged me to go for it.

I watched him around these very wealthy people and marvelled at how at ease he was. He was being himself, he wasn't putting on airs and graces, he was just being himself and was completely comfortable with that.

When I look back now, he had only reached Year 11 or maybe Year 12 at the local state school; considering these people had attended highly prestigious schools and universities, it showed how hard he had worked to feel comfortable amongst them.

He always strove to be better but was at ease wherever he was – I wanted that!

I decided the first thing I would tackle was travel.

I set a date and saved every penny I could to go to the United States. I was supposed to go with a girlfriend, but she wanted to put off the departure date. I had a date set and I was sticking to it. I think I was too scared not to stick to it in case it didn't happen!

So off I went to the U.S. on my own. My boyfriend organized some places for me to stay and I also did a Trek America and had the best time of my life. When I did the Trek we spent a lot of time camping in National Parks and it was there I decided I wanted to be a (ta da!!!) Park Ranger.

I came home and told my boyfriend my dream.

BUT I had to go back to school. I was now 20 and hadn't been to school for six years and I was petrified because I still thought I was dumb.

I decided (with his relentless encouragement) to start with some correspondence modules of the course I needed to do, to see if I thought I could pass it.

My first assignment came back with red pen all over it and to say I was devastated was a mass understatement. My boyfriend said, "Well you just have to do it again."

What?? I HATE having to do ANYTHING twice!

With his help I worked on the assignment and sent it back again and it came back with a 'B'. You couldn't wipe the grin off my face and after that there was no stopping me.

Later that year I decided I would apply for a place in the fulltime course, which was an Associate Diploma of Applied Science in Natural Resource Management.

The day the letter arrived it was just like the movies – I couldn't open it.

I waited for my boyfriend to get home and open it and I was in!! I was sooo excited and so was he; while I had always had my doubts, he always believed I could do it.

I started school the following year and in one of my first classes my worst fears were realized. One of the first subjects I encountered was land surveying and this meant trigonometry.

Not something I had learned in my three years at high school!

I sat through the whole class feeling completely stupid, filled with a sense of dread. I was going to fail. I didn't understand one word of what was said; it was mortifying and soul destroying.

I made a decision there and then that if I were to pass this thing I needed to ask for help. This was big for someone used to faking it!

I went to my lecturer's office at lunchtime and let him know my situation and that I was struggling badly. He told me this was not a problem and to come and see him at lunch times and he would talk me through it. The first lunchtime we started and he asked if I understood what he had shown me.

Nope! "OK, then let's go back a bit further… do you understand that?"

Nope! "OK, let's just start from the beginning."

Now that sounds more like it ☺

This man spent three weeks of lunch breaks with me, helping me understand and become confident with trigonometry.

Conquering that thing was like winning a gold medal.

The feeling of pride and fulfilment that came over me knowing I could learn something like that was like nothing else.

I will never, ever forget that feeling or my lecturer's kindness and generosity and I know for sure this has helped me further along the path I am still traveling today.

FLYING HIGH...

At the time my boyfriend and I lived in South Gippsland in Victoria and my school was in Frankston, about 90 minutes away! While my boyfriend was overseas, I had started learning to fly.

I wanted to give it a try while he was away so if I was crap at it he wouldn't need to know I had even tried – old habits die hard! Anyway I was good at it, very good at it, and got a job at the local airfield to help pay for my flying lessons and when I told him, he was as pleased as punch.

I was a bit of a thrill seeker in general and even more so in the air. I would often get a call across the flight radio "Hotel Alfa Tango no steep turns in the training area" – doh!

There were days when I would drive 90 minutes from Korumburra (in South Gippsland) to Frankston, have a flying lesson on the way at Tooradin, go to school for the day, drive back home and then work a shift at the local pub.

School holidays were spent doing work experience in the forestry town of Powelltown while all of my straight-out-of-high-school classmates (all male except one) partied! I would do work experience during the week, work at the pub over the weekend, as well as do my shift at the airfield, and squeeze in time for my flying lessons.

It was a very full-on time but I loved every second of it knowing I was becoming more of the me I knew I wanted to become.

Our graduation ceremony is a day I will never forget.

It was held at Melbourne's Art Centre and my Mum came with me. I had passed everything and then some. I achieved some of the highest marks in the class. I was so proud! This is what I had wanted for years.

Then one of the proudest moments of my life happened!

In his address to the parents and graduating students, the Head Lecturer started talking about me!

Me!!

About my achievements, about my guts and determination to pass! I hadn't realized that my (what I now know were extraordinary) efforts were being noticed. All of the driving, the working over the holidays while everyone else was partying, having two jobs and flying, plus all of the challenges that I had had to overcome having left school so young!

He spoke about it all, and while I was proud of being able to conquer this thing called education, I was even prouder of my courage and determination to achieve.

This is a lesson that has never left me and it is why I value work ethic over talent every day of the week, because I know I started with less than nothing and worked my way through.

It was quite a surreal moment having my Mum sit beside me whilst all of this was being said.

I was proud of what I had done and who I had become along the way, but I also wanted to say to my Mum, "SEE! I COULD DO IT, I AM SMART!"

Sadly my boyfriend and I broke up just before I graduated so he wasn't there to hear any of this. As I write this today, I realize he absolutely should have been there, despite everything – my graduation success was as much his as it was mine.

Now I am able to speak of how much he helped me and helped shape who I would become, even at 16, but sadly back then I was so full of insecurity and anger that I wasn't able to see this or if I saw it, I was too selfish and caught up in myself to acknowledge it.

I don't have regrets in my life – you make the best choices based on the information you have at the time, but I have to say I wish I could thank him now.

When I finished my course I was frustrated to see that any jobs in the Department of Conservation and Environment (as it was known then) were going to people who 'knew people' or people already employed by the government in another department.

I never ended up using that qualification, but it didn't matter! It was enough that I had done it and done it well! And it marked a significant turning point in my life.

It was about this time that Taekwondo entered my life. And for good and bad so did my first husband!

SOME MORE (EXCELLENT) GOOD
AND SOME BAD...
FINDING MY PLACE IN THE WORLD...

Taekwondo and I clicked from the second I started. You could say we found each other and there was no looking back.

THIS was my thing.

This is what I was put on earth to do, and while the journey was a hard one, an emotional one, a physically demanding one, I wouldn't change a second of it! Because much of the last 22 years of my life has been shaped in one way or another by Taekwondo.

When I first started training I liked to think I was a bit of a natural, I'm not sure that was the case but I was very zealous! I was committed to doing this for life... but I was in a rush.

I had my black belt in around two years because I 'double graded' most gradings and I was training seven days a week, including training as part of the State team and training under our Head Instructor, Mr Chang, at Frankston every Saturday morning.

I wanted to know everything and do everything perfectly from Day One. I would go hell for leather and it did not always end well. I often had plenty of bruises (both to my body and my ego) to show for it!

Very early on, I started assisting my instructor. He later became my husband, and then later again, my ex-husband! I look back at him as fitting two roles – one as an inspirational and amazing instructor – and one as my less-than-perfect ex-husband. As time went on the line became blurry, but for the most part I look back on the times he was my instructor with fondness, as a husband… not so much!

Anyway I was assisting the classes from about six months into my training and I loved it. I took to instructing like a duck to water and I felt immediately comfortable in that role. I loved helping others achieve their goals, it filled me with immense satisfaction and sat nicely alongside my natural desire to be bossy.

I started competing in full contact sparring competitions very early on as well, I think I had my first fight about six months into training.

The build-up and the training for that first fight was a killer. We were a nice sized club and a lot of us wanted to compete in sparring. My instructor had a very impressive competition career and this was his passion, and his knowledge was passed on to us without a second thought.

We had a great team of competitors and we trained the house down. I have a light frame and stand at 165cm. My weight went from a slightly chubby and very soft 59kg when I started, to a lean and muscular 46kg when I was training for my first black belt fight; around two years into my training. It was intense!

We trained at 5am Monday, Wednesday and Friday mornings, as well as our regular classes at night five times a week. My instructor and I also trained on Saturdays at Frankston with our Korean Head Instructor, as well as State Team Training on Sundays.

I did this even after Cody was born, about four years into my training (he would come along in his pram) – it was full on!

We were always soooo sore!

We were sore from training, sore from contact injuries, sore from niggling injuries, but there was no way we wanted to miss a training session.

THE L WORD...

I suffered very badly from pre-fight nerves – I mean it was so bad I wouldn't speak to anyone for a week before a fight and if forced to answer a question it was usually answered in the form of a grunt! I didn't have to worry about making weight because I struggled to eat.

The nerves weren't about being hurt, but about not winning, I still struggle to use that 'L' word that describes not winning!

My first fight was one which everyone in the club expected me to win, but long story short... I didn't! I was so ashamed; I can't even describe the pain of it. I look back now and I can see it wasn't as bad as it felt at the time, but it still bites even today!

The girl I fought that day was from another club associated with ours, so we had sparred together on Saturday mornings. She had been training for about two years to my six months, but hadn't graded to go up in belts.

On the day of the fight I got white line fever and punched her in the face three times.

Good if I was boxing, but not so good in Taekwondo. In competition Taekwondo this is a no-no – you can kick the face and body, but you cannot punch the face.

Long story short I lost by 1 point after having 3 points taken off me. How rude!

The poor girl would have wondered what the hell hit her!

Thankfully I learned much from that first fight.

I also got to experience the awful, awful taste of eating humble pie as I headed back to the club a loser! There I said it! The dreaded 'L' word.

I actually couldn't face going back to training the first night after the competition because I was soooo embarrassed.

I was very touched when one of the girls from training called me and told me they missed me; I had done well and they wanted to see me back at training the next night.

I imagine my instructor had something to do with that phone call, but it meant a lot just the same. I had a medal, but it wasn't a winning medal, so it took some doing for me to put up my one and only Bronze Medal at my Taekwondo school years later! Humility is clearly the Traditional Precept I still have yet to fully grasp.

I learned then that the only person putting this massive weight of pressure on me was me. The others all respected me: win, lose or draw. That was it meant to be part of a team, something completely foreign to me.

A lot of us didn't win that day but we gave it a red-hot go!

After that competition a few people decided tournament fighting was no longer for them but they continued training and were there to cheer us on.

Out of all of the students who started when I did, as far as I know, I am the only one still training. As far as competition went, I had unfinished business and I was not going to "L… L… L… NOT win again"!

WINNERS ARE GRINNERS…

My next fight was as a blue belt and there was a girl in my weight division who was a bit of a worry. The day of my first comp I had watched her smash another girl's nose across her face with an axe kick. As soon as we worked out that she would be in my division for my next competition, we constantly trained to avoid axe kicks, to ensure I finished the fight with all of the parts of my face in the right spot!

Comp day came and I won two or three fights to the final and fought 'axe kick' girl somewhere early on. Happy to report she didn't land one axe kick and I won the division that day and made my first State team.

I went to nationals and won my weight division against some much bigger girls, because they had put a couple of weight divisions together to create a bigger draw for us.

The girl I met in the final was about 8kg heavier and taller than me and she kept punching my chest above the protector and I felt like I was being hit with a hammer.

It was my last fight for the day and it was getting late.

We had weighed in at 6am, I had my first fight around 10.30am, my next fight was around 5pm and then this last fight was around 9.30 at night. I was exhausted and a long wait between matches means all of the bumps and bruises acquired over the earlier part of the day haunt you and just make you feel rotten. To be honest I just wanted to pick up my bat and ball and go home – I was over it.

During the fight I realized I was the last fight of the day and mine was the only match running at that time. I looked up to see many of the Victorian team in the front stand cheering me on. I was so tired and beat up but it lifted me, there was no way I was going to not win with everyone watching! I won, and afterwards it was like I had just woken up, I had all the energy in the world and was pumped. Winning does that to you ☺

The after parties when we went interstate were always so funny. Everyone was bruised and limping and had ice packs strapped to them. Everyone liked to glam up for the events, but that just made it all the more funny. A band of glamorous, skinny, walking wounded. It still makes me smile when I remember it.

Those nights were awesome.

Everyone had been dieting and training hard and it was time to cut loose. All of the Korean Head Instructors attended the dinners and I loved spending time with them. After the Head Instructors left, everyone let their hair down and for the most part even if you had been fighting someone that day, that night you were mates. Club rivalries were put on hold and everyone just had a ball.

Fighting is a very intimate thing.

Here you are trying to knock each other out so you don't need to go the distance. Knowing the less time in the ring you have the better, because you have other fights coming up and you will be less banged up.

Before the fight you usually stay away from each other. You bow at the start and then when the ref calls "Sijak" it is game on. For the next little while it is all about winning. Afterwards you bow and go shake the hand of your opponent's coach as is compulsory. But you also do something that is not compulsory. You hug your opponent and you mean it.

You have both been through the same thing, and whether you have won or not you still respect the person you just fought. And only the two of you know what you just went through and will relive the same memories, albeit from a different perspective for many years to come.

That is one of the things I love most about this sport and if it didn't have this very human side I wouldn't have been as drawn to it as I was.

My first black belt fight was six weeks after I had earned it. This was SCARY! In my division there were two very strong competitors who had both been overseas with one medalling and one the current National Champion.

I think I had three fights that day and the final was against the current National Champ. She was known for this loud screech. We "gihap" when we kick or score (this is the noise like a yell you hear in sparring) but hers was ridiculous.

I can remember in the first round she did her screech and I just looked at her like "Are you for real?!" and that gave her exactly what she wanted! As I was busy pulling a face and thinking I was cool, she scored a beautiful cracking roundhouse kick point. I was open and she took it. I was fuming with myself.

In spite of that bad start, I went on to win my first ever black belt fight, and against the current national champ to boot. I was one happy girl.

I could talk about competing and competition training for days on end, but I'll stop here, except to say that those days were some of the fondest memories I have of my training.

I sometimes find it hard to accept that I will never have those days again and that that part of my life is now in the past. If I think about it too much, it can dim the future knowing that type of training and winning is not going to happen anymore. There is nothing that will match the highs of competition and competition training, and everything else seems second best.

PAYING IT FORWARD…

When I finished competing, I started coaching my own students in competition and that really does come a very close second to competing myself. Knowing I can give my students the same joy, and help to make the same memories for them, is priceless for me. It is almost equally as fulfilling as my own competing, that's for sure. And far less painful!

My instructor was incredible. Enough time and distance has now passed to wash away any lingering anger that remained from him also being my ex-husband.

Now that I have been instructing in my own Taekwondo schools for many years I can remember how special an atmosphere he created. He also created very strong minds and strong bodies. He was super fit, fast, strong and powerful and we were in awe watching him. We ate up the stories from his own training and overseas trips as a member of the National team.

I truly believe I had the best instructor around. He was able to extract the best from me, whilst also teaching me how to get the best from myself. He taught me how to love hard training; how to train so hard I had to vomit.

As part of my training I used to love running stairs – well, actually I love it NOW, I don't think I loved it so much then!! We lived in Inverloch along the coast in Victoria and there are some awesome sets of stairs on the way down to the beaches. One is called Eagles Nest. The other is called Shack Bay.

My instructors favourite training ground at one point was Eagles Nest. These stairs are a killer. It is a long, long way from top to bottom; the stairs are sometimes nothing more than dirt and sleepers, then there are bits with no steps and just an incline.

Imagine you are running straight up a cliff, like a cut cat, and dodging water courses and uneven ground, and your lungs are screaming.

Running stairs is THE BEST training you will ever do, but it is just nuts.

Shack Bay was safer because the wooden steps are evenly placed but it could be slippery in the wet. At Shack Bay my instructor/husband could watch me the whole way up and would sit at the top yelling at me. I remember one day I was tired, sore and just over training. I was sulking before we even got to the stairs.

My warm-up was always running, then sprints on the beach, which I HATED.

On the way I said, "If the tide is in and the sand is soft, I'm not running." Well, the tide was in and the sand was soft, and after arguing and being told not to speak to my instructor like that (I thought I was talking to my husband!) I started jogging in the soft sand. It was all too much in my tired and emotional state, and I cracked it.

I threw my runners off and yelled, "If I have to run in soft sand I'm not wearing shoes!" He told me to stop being a baby, get my shoes on so I wouldn't cut my feet open a week before Nationals, and get on with it. I sucked it up, put my shoes on and got on with it.

I laugh at it now, because he must have been wetting himself laughing, watching me throw a hissy fit like a spoiled brat. But man, I was cranky.

In time I would go and do those stairs just for fun. I roped in some of the mums from Cody's play group to come and play as well, and those stairs were a solid part of my training three or four times a week.

I laugh again when I think back to the first time the mums met me at the stairs. One mum had a matching scrunchie and socks (it was the 90s!) and a face full of make-up. After about two sets she had to lie down because she was going to faint. Not funny for her, but pretty funny for me!

At my peak I could run thirty flights of Shack Bay Stairs and eat it up.

Recently one of my students and I headed to Shack Bay stairs to do a training session and I was anxious and excited at the same time. That feeling you get when you know something is going to hurt… a lot!

We took it in turns up and down, so we got a small rest break between flights, but we did 37 flights before we ran out of time.

Nowadays I still like to get down to Inverloch and run them whenever I can.

AND NOW THE UGLY!
WHAT SHOULD HAVE BEEN VERY GOOD...

My marriage was full of highs and lows. Eventually there were way too many lows and we were destroying each other.

We met in 1990 and separated in 1997. It was not a very long time, but our marriage affected us both deeply in many ways for a very long time, and I am sure it still does to some extent. What should have been very good ended up being very bad.

Once we had separated I discovered I was pregnant with my second child, my daughter Chloe.

So there I was: pregnant, living two hours from my family with a small toddler and on my own. That was the start of a few very difficult years.

If I could describe those years in a word I would have to say it was devastating.

I had separated from the person I was meant to be with for the rest of my life and who I fell in love with very, very deeply.

Some of the lowest points were during a very, very nasty family court battle, where I felt under siege for a very long time, never knowing what was coming next.

Often I would be getting ready to go and instruct at my Taekwondo school and the mail would arrive with the tell-tale logo from the Court or my husband's solicitor, with some accusation or request that would feel like a kick in the guts. But I would have to suck it up and go teach classes and inspire my students.

I felt ashamed of the fact I was teaching my martial art pregnant and without a husband. I felt I was not being the person I needed to be, to set the example I wanted to set. This hurt me so much because leading by example and living with integrity are core values that mean a lot to me. I felt like I was letting my students down and placing the parents in an awkward position having to explain the situation to my students, their children. I guess this was residual from my earlier life when I seemed to always feel some sort of shame.

There was also the time I went for my pre-natal check-up before I went to teach Taekwondo, only to be told my baby (Chloe) had died at around 19 weeks and that I would have to deliver the baby the following week.

I went and taught classes that night then attended a tournament the following day (as a coach) and all the while I was dealing with the fact I had a dead baby inside of me.

I went back for another scan on the following Monday only to be told that it had been an incorrect diagnosis and in fact Chloe was alive and well. But the sadness, anger, fear and sense of loss I experienced for those few days would never leave me.

Chloe's birth was not good.

My husband was there in body, but couldn't have cared less about the pain I was in – a very, very different experience to our son Cody's birth when he was so wonderful and cried at the pain I was in, and with happiness at the birth of his son, our first child.

After the birth of Chloe, I begged him to bring 2-year-old Cody in to see us, but he took his sweet time and it was days before I saw my little boy, I was an emotional wreck.

I was allowed out of the hospital for dinner one night, and he picked me up and took me out for dinner and it ended in a very bad argument. I was hysterical by the time I got back to the hospital – I'm not a hysterical kind of girl but hormones are a bitch!

I saw the look on the nurse's face when she saw me, and then I caught her scowling at my husband. It made me feel so pathetic and worthless because I could see pity on her face and as I said before, I don't do pity.

A while after this I was also a witness for the prosecution in separate proceedings against my husband that ultimately sent him to jail. This was rough, really rough! But I got through it, knowing I had to do what I knew to be right. I had to stand up, even though the last thing I needed was more court time and drama in my life.

One shining lesson from that whole experience is something I'll never forget – so simple, but powerful.

I was stressing out about testifying and being perfect on the stand. The police said to me, "You don't have to try to win this thing for us, you just have to tell the truth."

Here I was, thinking I was going to make or break the case (not much of an ego!). Thinking I had to be perfect, and wearing the weight of that was unbearable. When really I was a small part of a much bigger picture, and all I had to do was tell the truth.

Hell, I could do that!

Telling my children their father had gone to prison, and answering the question, "Do you think daddy should be in jail?" were not easy things to deal with, but we got through it.

That was probably the only time the kids saw me cry, but we cried together. They knew that while I did believe he needed to serve time in jail, I was sad for him, and scared for him, and despite everything, still cared for him.

My ex had met someone new, I'm guessing just prior to the birth of my daughter, and was never around when I needed help. I was a single mum with a new baby, a toddler, a Taekwondo school to run and no family support.

I received no financial support for the kids so I had to keep working and babysitters had to become a way of life for our small family.

I was tough and I was resilient and I got on with doing what I had to do.

I was also lucky enough to have made a very wonderful friend called Carolyn, who helped me get through the toughest bits. She was always there ready to do whatever she could and she cared very much for my children.

Without her it would have been an absolute nightmare for sure.

I look back on those years now and don't know how the hell I did it. But I did, and while those years fill me with sadness if I let myself go there, they also made me one tough cookie.

After more than a decade of fighting, followed by a decade of silence, I invited my ex-husband back into my life and the lives of my children and I now have a wonderful friendship with him, as do the kids, and it feels awesome to co-parent as we should have been able to all along.

The healing from this was immense.

It is wonderful to have my instructor back and to be able to share the good memories and I know it was good for the kids too.

The years between 1997 and the early 2000s, life was a rollercoaster.

In 1999 I married again, to a man who loved me and my kids. I didn't love him, but I knew he would be stable and not cheat on me. I liked him a lot, but I should never have married him.

I thought I was over my ex and just wanted to put all of the mess behind me and get on with life.

But very quickly I realized I had settled and it ate at me every day. I was miserable.

Eleven months later we separated. It was awful. I hurt him, it was a mess, and it was my fault.

I heard he ran his car into a tree not long after our separation and the guilt nearly killed me. He survived, and recovered, and today he is happily married with his own children. He still sees my children from time to time – something I am forever grateful for, because he truly deserves to be happy.

IT ALL STARTS WITH TRAINING...

In my life I have made many mistakes. I have done many things I wish I hadn't. I have behaved in ways I wish I could take back.

I wish when I was younger I'd had the wisdom I have now, but it doesn't work that way does it! What is done is done, and I know better now and am wiser for the experience.

What I have done is to look at all of my life experiences (and there are many), and I have decided that all of those experiences, the good ones and the bad ones, make me who I am today for good or for bad.

I am happy to say that I really like who I am today.

I love parts of who I was over the years, because I can now look back fondly at the young woman who crashed and bashed her way through life, taking her challenges head-on, trying to get ahead in life the best way she knew how.

Throughout it all though the one thing that has remained constant is this...

When I was in peak shape and training as I should be EVERYTHING ELSE fell into place.

During my divorce and messy family court stuff, if I stopped training at intensity and being grounded in my Taekwondo training because I was overanxious and stressed, the wheels fell off everything. When I made the decision to smash myself back into shape, everything else started to become more positive and flow the way I wanted (and needed) it to.

If I am struggling for inspiration in my business, it is usually because work has taken over and I'm not training the way I should. Every time I have had a business idea, or new idea for an adventure that I am excited about, it has come from being in a peak state of fitness and training hard in Taekwondo, which always grounds me.

When you are training as you should, everything is firing on all cylinders and you are filled with energy and vitality. The small things that bug you evaporate, and the big things that challenge you, become something you know you can overcome.

In this state you just want to go for it, grab life by the throat and make things happen.

In essence, it ALL starts with your training.

There are many parallels between life and training – where you find a powerful training message it is usually a metaphor for life and vice versa.

The two are linked and there is no separating them.

Whenever I hear of a woman struggling with divorce I go out of my way to encourage her to start training and get in shape. I tell her nothing bad will ever come from getting in shape, and many, many good things are likely to happen as a result of being fit, strong and healthy through good training.

It is always emotional for me to see how much this is so, to see a woman go from a place of total despair to feeling so empowered she knows there is nothing she can't achieve, nothing she cannot overcome.

This is what this book is all about – finding your indomitable spirit and getting to a place of knowing that you can do, be, and have everything you truly want in life if you are willing to work for it.

I also want to challenge your mindset about the way you go about your training and if you're concerned about your weight, how you deal with losing that weight.

My promise to you is that by the time you finish reading this book you will be ready to roll your sleeves up and do whatever it takes to find your own bulletproof confidence and train your way to a kickass body AND enjoy the ride!

PART TWO:

BULLETPROOF CONFIDENCE

HOW DID I GET HERE?

The number one cause of frustration amongst the women in my world is their constant struggle with their unfulfilled potential.

That nagging, burning, sickening hole deep inside that reminds you of all the things you've said or thought you would achieve but until now haven't been able to.

Usually this unfulfilled potential falls into any combination of these three categories:

- Your Physical Self

- Your Personal Achievements

- Your ability to live the life you really, truly want

Unfulfilled potential takes up a lot of mental space and energy that could and should be used for more productive and positive things.

If you did a tally of the amount of time you spent each day agonising over your shortcomings and beating yourself up over them, I'm pretty sure it would shock you.

With all of these thoughts filling your head day in day out, I think it is fair to say that the noise level in your head is probably quite deafening. Moreover that deafening noise is taking up valuable space and creating the sort of nagging overwhelm that paralyses you and stops you from getting anywhere fast.

To quiet the noise and fill the void you may be constantly looking for the next big, bright, shiny distraction, but this continual searching just adds to the mess… and deep down you know this to be true.

The world around us has become sloppy, undisciplined and fraught with franticness. Temptation is all around, things that we used to pay lots of money for and cherish dearly are now throw-away objects discarded at the first hint of the next best thing. These days most families cannot even sit together at a dinner table without at least two mobile phones sitting front and centre.

We have a short attention span and self-discipline is at an all-time low, particularly when it comes to the way we treat out bodies and our minds.

Our bodies are fed on a diet of sugar and fat and our minds are fed on a toxic diet of messages delivered from every angle; magazines are filled with recycled rubbish not fit for human consumption, and social media, commercial television and radio all deliver their fair share of toxic messages on a daily basis.

This overwhelm and noise has taken a toll on women and as a result something has had to give. We have become mentally soft and so have our bodies; motivation and energy levels are depleted and confidence and self-esteem are at an all-time low.

Chances are you are caught up in what I call the "Monday Merry Go Round", where every Monday you vow to start again and do it right this week, you set your standards unattainably high and by Wednesday it all falls apart and yet again you tell yourself that you will start again next Monday . Maybe now you have also started to ask the question "How the hell did I get here?"

Am I right or am I right??

I know you are highly intelligent and have a truckload of knowledge about what and how you should be doing things to bridge the gap between who you are now and who you really know you can be physically and emotionally.

Deep down you know there is no magic bullet and there are no quick fixes that offer sustainable results, because if there were you would have discovered them by now after all your years of trying.

I hope that by picking up and purchasing this book you are ready to roll up your sleeves and begin to do what your gut has been telling you to do for years and that is to start to do some real work and get clear on what you really truly want from all areas of your life. The aim of this book is to encourage you to create your own plan of action and the discipline to follow through until the end and let me tell you right now, this is exactly what will bridge that gap you have been trying so desperately trying to fill for years and years.

I came to martial arts 22 years ago after growing up exposed to domestic violence, sexual abuse and poverty and I know first-hand that the quickest and most efficient way to build self-esteem, bullet-proof confidence and a kickass body is within the martial arts environment, utilising martial arts training and philosophies.

I know this because I have lived it and I know this because I have helped countless other women, either through martial arts training, martial arts philosophies or both, achieve the bulletproof confidence they need to courageously step up and grab the life they truly want for themselves.

When we start this journey I always begin with training and nutrition, because if your body does not look and function the way you want it to, you are behind the 8 ball EVERY SINGLE TIME – NO EXCEPTIONS.

The way our physical self shows up in the world is a reflection of what is going on inside. If you are overweight and tired this is a direct result of the way you are living your life and that includes how you are feeding both your mind and your body.

There is no hiding from this fact, what you are doing to your body and mind on a daily basis is what looks straight back at you in the mirror every single morning as a constant reminder.

The opposite is also true; when you look smoking hot and have energy to burn this too is a reflection of what you are feeding your body and mind.

No one gets to be fit and healthy by accident, it is a direct result of the things you feed your mind and body. This includes skinny women who look good with their clothes on! Believe it or not, you can be thin and unhealthy so don't be deceived by looks alone. What you want is to be fit, healthy, lean and strong – only then will you feel as good as you look and have the energy and vibrancy you need to live this life you truly want.

Being fit, healthy, energetic and vibrant and feeling confident in the way you look puts you in the perfect state for pursuing the life of your dreams.

The very fact you are reading this book leads me to believe you already know the feeling I am talking about because I am guessing this is not your first rodeo!

Chances are you have already experienced being in that state of flow once before; probably even more than once, but consistency over time has eluded you and you are frustrated with yourself because you just can't seem to maintain this state – the state you know is key to living the life and achieving the dreams you have for yourself.

This is precisely why training like a black belt and developing Bulletproof Confidence and everything that involves is exactly what you need right now.

The traditional tenets of Self-Control, Excellence, Perseverance, Courage and Indomitable Spirit (just to name a few) will help set the foundation you need to get on with the job of creating the life you truly want and creating a cracking body to take with you on the journey.

TAKING FROM THE MARTIAL ARTS PRINCIPLES

Whenever I teach a self- defence seminar, I always encourage the participants to seriously consider taking up regular martial arts classes. I tell them, "Nothing bad ever came from regular training and gaining your black belt" and the same can be said for adopting the principles of Martial Arts into your daily life.

Who doesn't want to be able to regularly exercise self-control when the need arises? And I can't think of a single example where excellence is not worth pursuing, nor can I see how becoming courageous and resilient would ever be considered a waste of time.

The way you behave in your daily life determines how and where you end up. By embracing and introducing each of the principles into your daily life you are setting the foundation to live every day in a way that allows you to walk through life with your head held high, knowing you not only hold yourself to a higher standard but you also meet that standard a good portion of the time.

There is no greater sense of peace or accomplishment than when you can look everyone you meet square in the eye, or can walk into any room filled to the brim with people without hesitation, or take on any challenge handed to you head on, or say YES to any opportunity presented to you NOW because you know you are worthy and you know you are ready.

A strong sense of worthiness, coupled with preparedness, will propel you far in life. Think about all of the times you said "No" to an opportunity because you weren't ready or because you didn't feel good enough. I know this first hand. Leaving school at 14 and growing up with the experiences I did left me feeling extremely unworthy, and looking back I can see that while I had the fire in my belly and the desire to achieve great things, even as a teenager, what held me back was not feeling 'ready' because I needed to do, be, and have more to feel worthy enough. I believed that only when I felt worthy, would I be ready.

The problem with this as you have probably already experienced is that the goal posts keep shifting and there is never any definitive moment when you feel as though you are suddenly ready or worthy, so you can't rely on waiting for these feelings of worthiness and readiness to appear.

Worthiness and preparedness are by-products of living these Martial Arts Principles on a daily basis. As you work through this book you will notice how this process changes you and how differently people begin to respond to you.

Interesting things happens to the people around you when you decide to live your life with a deep sense of personal integrity and not all of them feel good. You will notice the negative people in your life become noticeably more negative and even derisive of your attitude and decisions, and often these individuals fall by the wayside. You will also notice you start to attract people into your world who share your values, beliefs and passions, and you may even discover a deeper level of connection with people you already know superficially.

Good attracts good, strong attracts strong, and who you attract into your life will be a reflection of who **you are** in your own life.

If all of a sudden you notice yourself surrounded by superficial, lazy, negative people there is a good chance YOU too have become superficial, lazy and negative. This is often a tough wake-up call, but to recognise your shortcomings, whatever they are, means you now see them and can get on with the job of becoming the person you can be proud of. The person who can look anyone square in the eye or confidently walk into a crowded room or say "Yes" to any opportunity that knocks on your door.

We all want to feel proud of who we are and the things we do with our lives and we have all felt the consequences of not doing so; feelings of inadequacy, insecurity or worse and living in a body we hate that cannot do the things we urge it to do. This is not living, this is existing, this is biding time till you die.

Practicing Martial Arts Principles on a daily basis is not the easiest path to walk, but it is highly rewarding and just like with regular training in Martial Arts, you will never regret it and nothing bad will ever come of it. So make the decision today to live your life differently, from the way you think about the smallest and most mundane things, to the big stuff like who you allow to spend time in your world or how you choose to make your living.

Finding a strong role model with depth, substance, ethics and integrity, along with your specific beliefs and values, can be difficult (if not impossible) so here is a thought… be your own hero; be the person you can look up to, depend upon and be inspired by. Create a specific and systematic set of behaviours for yourself (based on the principles) that you follow day in day out, and become that person for yourself. By doing this you will also find that along the way you will inadvertently become that person for the people around you.

I never set out to be an inspiration or role model for anyone; all I was trying to do was be the best possible version of myself I could become. I did it consistently, and along the way I almost subconsciously began to set higher and higher standards for myself and it was important to me to rise to these standards again and again. Because I was so passionate and excited about the changes I could see in myself from making some small but consistent changes in my thinking and approach, I started to notice the people around me who could also benefit from changing their thinking and behaviour. These people were seeking me out to help them become stronger and more confident, fitter and leaner. To this day I love nothing more than helping women discover their best self, which is all I want for you too.

Ok, let's get stuck into the principles and philosophies that will change your life!

When writing this book it seemed that my favourite topic was ME, so you will find plenty of examples throughout this book, based on my own learnings that I hope will help you understand what the hell I'm talking about.

WORKING YOUR WAY TO
A BLACK BELT MINDSET

In my style of Taekwondo our bank ranking goes like this:

WHITE BELT

YELLOW BELT

BLUE BELT

RED BELT

BLACK BELT

Each of the coloured belts (yellow, blue, black) has three stripes to be earned before moving on to the next colour.

Students move progressively through each belt level and each of the colours – white, yellow, blue, red and black – has its own significance that I have related to your own journey towards achieving a black belt attitude for life.

WHITE signifies the beginning, that the student has no previous knowledge.

The greatest gift you can give yourself right now is to come to this as a white belt. Forget what you already know (just for now) and clear your mind of the clutter you have accumulated over the years that is taking up space in your mind and creating confusion and overwhelm.

Just let it all go, safe in the knowledge you will be able to come back and select only the very best and most useful bits of information you have locked away in amongst all of the faff.

Start with a fresh mind, a clean slate and only fill it with what you really need and know to be right for you. Make conscious and selective choices about what you let into your life from here.

White = clarity, simplicity, uncomplicated, uncluttered

YELLOW signifies the laying of the foundation.

Once you have dumped all of the guff and you are laser clear on what you want your life to be about from here on in, this is where you begin.

Look at what you already know is useful that will help you achieve this path you are now on. Here is where you create that specific and systematic set of behaviours for yourself to follow day in day out, knowing that this is what will guide you towards becoming the person you truly wish to be.

Yellow = only adding what is true and right for you, establishing strong behaviours and habits.

BLUE signifies the maturing of the student's learning.

Once the foundations have been laid and you have spent some time living this way, you then begin to fall into a rhythm where you can clearly begin to see what fits and what does not, and be able to make decisions based on this more readily. You are now beginning to really understand what works for you and how to apply it and at the same time how to avoid what does not work for you.

This stage is also where the novelty starts to wear off and the hard work begins.

Blue = discernment, keeping what works and discarding the rest, the work starts.

RED signifies danger and caution.

In the belt ranking system of life, red is complacency. Here is where you begin to take some shortcuts and things start to unravel. In Taekwondo many students have come very close to earning their black belt only to quit at red belt level. This is where you need to dig deep and push through to the other side, knowing there will be great rewards for your effort.

Red = time to be disciplined and diligent to stay the path.

BLACK is the opposite of white signifying a level of proficiency.

In Taekwondo students are very surprised to learn that once you get your black belt this is when the real learning begins, and that everything achieved up until this point has just been establishing the basics, particularly in mindset. Many people think that a black belt means you have made it and consequently many people stop training once they achieve this level. They are completely missing the point by thinking that the attainment of the black belt is the achievement.

I have always told my students (as my instructor told me and his instructor told him before that, and no doubt Mr Chang's Instructor told him exactly the same thing back in Korea many, many years ago) if you stop training once you get to black belt then you **were** once a black belt, if you don't train anymore, you are no longer a black belt, you simply were one once upon a time.

The same is true for anything you do in life. So long as you eat clean and train hard on a consistent basis you can call yourself an athlete (recreational or otherwise) and the way your body looks will reflect this. When you no longer eat this way or train regularly, you were once an athlete but are no longer and again your body will reflect this too.

To maintain the level of black belt or to progress forward through the black belt rankings (2nd dan through to 10th dan) you cannot simply stay the same, you need to be constantly learning and growing and improving. If you are not moving forwards you can be certain you are moving backwards because we never, ever remain in suspension.

Once you have mastered your new way of living, have created the body and life you desire and have developed your black belt attitude, without continued work it will all be lost. The work begins now and this is where you use all of the lessons you learned along the way to help you stay the path and help you get back on it should you wander off for a little while.

This is the essence of the black belt, remaining a lifelong student and understanding that the job is never done; it is a lifelong endeavour that you embrace.

Black = high level of proficiency and lifelong dedication.

I'm sure you can see how your past attempts fit in to the ranking system above.

Which belt level did you quit at last time?

Are you ready now to meet the challenge head on and push through?

I hope that knowing you are human and that this is a natural process for many will help encourage you to put aside past failures and aim for your personal black belt.

SEASONS, HARD AND SOFT

Nobody is perfect and nobody expects you to be perfect. Humans are flawed beings and whilst intellectually we know what we should be doing and how we should be doing it, sometimes we just don't.

We humans fluctuate like the seasons; we have our summers, our autumns our winters and our springs. The more we know ourselves, the better able we are to manage our seasons.

We are also hard and soft – sometimes we need to be hard on ourselves and other times we need to be soft; from a training perspective seasons of hard and soft are crucial for improvement.

It took me until my very late 30s to figure out that it isn't possible to maintain absolute peak fitness every day of the year, year in year out. This was me all hard and no soft and not acknowledging the need for seasons (base, build, peak, taper, perform, recover). It still bugs me that in my effort to train the house down day after day I was actually hindering my improvement.

I fought the notion of hard and soft and seasons day after day for two decades and would probably still be fighting it until this day had my (older) body not let me know in no uncertain terms that this was not possible. For years I was plagued by injury and it frustrated the hell out of me, but I still didn't listen to what everyone else was telling me: that not every single training session can be performed with gut busting intensity and that my body needed recovery time.

If I went in early to the dojang to do some solo training I had to get to the point of vomiting or it wasn't hard enough.

One day I headed into the dojang and my body was tired, my mind was tired and it was ridiculous to even entertain the thought of another training session. I figured that as I was there I may as well do something and I wanted to kick. So instead of pumping out 20 or 30 kicks in fast succession, I did sets of three and picked apart my technique (something I hadn't done in a long time). I smoothed out some techniques that had been bothering me and the improvements were significant. Now I always include some low intensity technique work as well as the higher intensity stuff when I train.

If I ran it was at flat out and over the years I found I never really improved my times, neither could I run any decent distance, because every session I kept trying to be faster. This was despite the fact that my clients were knocking ridiculous amounts of time off their runs because they were following the plans I had set them!

I know.... how ridiculous!

When I learned that not every run should be a flat out sprint I discovered that I could in fact run further than 3km. I even went to Paris to run the Paris Marathon for my 40th birthday. Running distance is not my thing but the knowledge that I could do it was amazing and all it took was one small adjustment; adding some soft.

What I want you to take from this is the understanding that we cannot and should not maintain peak fitness all year round BUT we do need to draw a line in the sand about what is acceptable in between and be diligent about working towards peak fitness at least four times a year so we keep our edge.

The following principles should weather all of the seasons, and when embraced daily the following will change your life forever.

THE PRINCIPLES

INDOMITABLE SPIRIT

Indomitable Spirit is probably the traditional tenet that resonates most for me. I have been a fighter one way or another all of my life beginning with my early childhood. Over the years, well before I even knew what Indomitable Spirit was, I refused to accept defeat in any area of my life nor would I allow anyone to 'conquer' or intimidate me.

The word indomitable means 'unconquerable' or impossible to defeat.

Spirit is the fire in your belly, your core gut level strength and determination to succeed.

You have probably heard the saying "It isn't the size of the dog in the fight but the size of the fight in the dog" and this too sums up indomitable spirit; it is winning against all of the odds and never saying die.

Whenever you struggle in any area of your life it is time to stoke that fire in your belly and strengthen your resolve to give it another crack.

A typical scenario for women (this may even be you?) who want to lose weight is this...

They have trained well and maintained good nutrition for one week then they get on the scales only to be devastated that all of the effort they put into practice for a whole week hasn't paid off, and so off they go to eat a muffin because it is just so unfair, and so the spiral begins.

OR

You have been training for a half marathon and in the lead up you become injured and have to pull out of the race. I have worked with enough female recreational athletes to know that this is always pretty devastating and one of two things happens. 1: The athlete is upset and annoyed but deals with the fact by knowing they can compete in that specific event next year. While they can't run they can swim, cycle, do weights, etc. to get them through being injured without losing the strength and fitness they have gained, or 2: The athlete finds themselves completely overwhelmed by the fact they can't race and if they can't race then what is the point of doing any training at all. They end up packing on the kilos and creating a frame of mind that starts the downward spiral and keeps them there for a long time.

Cultivating an Indomitable Spirit doesn't mean you don't have your moments of despair, but what it does mean is that you know you have no other option other than to pick yourself up, dust yourself off and continue to fight for your goals, regardless of the setbacks.

The biggest Taekwondo lesson I ever got in 'sucking it up' came very early on. I was yellow belt and had been training around six or seven months and our club entered its first competition. The competition was the State championships and it was the first fight for all of.

At the club I was sparring very well and the consensus was that I would win. The pressure I put on myself to win was enormous.

Was I worried about being knocked out or hurt? Hell no! All that I was worried about was that I would lose. To me that would mean total devastation.

Well they say "that what you fear, you create", and in this case it was right on the money! As I have mentioned before, in our style of Taekwondo the rules are you can kick or punch to the body, but only kick to the face (no punching the face). I got white line fever and punched the poor girl in the face not once, not twice, but three times! I lost by 1 point but had 3 points taken off me for punching her in the face.

I could not believe I had lost my fight; I was in shock and I was mortified; I did not want to go back to class the next night at all but I knew I had to, I knew I had to step up and finish what I started.

My next fight I was better prepared mentally (I don't think I could have been any better prepared physically), and I won my division which meant I made my first State team and from there I went on to win my first Nationals.

Don't worry, part of me wanted to quit after my defeat but there was no way I was going to let it happen. That defeat also taught me that 'nobody dies' when you don't win. I badly needed a good dose of perspective and that loss gave it to me and continues to serve as a lesson today.

Another AWFUL lesson I had the misfortune to experience, was handed out to me in the form of my first (and last!! – well at the time of writing!) Olympic Distance Triathlon. I remember many years ago (before triathlon was ever seriously on my radar) having a conversation with a fellow instructor, Steve, about triathlon. Steve competed regularly and I remember asking him, "What if you come last?" He said to me, "Someone always comes last and it is never you." I remembered this many years later when I did my first ever fun run and during each run or triathlon since it always served me well. In fact I repeat Steve's words often to the women who ask me the same thing.

Well once again what you fear you create. I did come last. Stone - motherless - last!

The swim leg freaked me out because the water was so black and there were apparently water snakes and eels in the lake. I thought I would be okay but I got about 300 metres into the 1500 metre swim and lost it. I tried hard to quiet my panic but after a number of attempts I called for the boat to come and pull me out. Turns out a lot of people were pulled out that day, but I'm pretty sure I was the only one to go on and finish the race.

Once I was in the boat I was told I could finish but I had to wait until everyone else had finished the swim. I was stuck in that boat for at least 30 minutes then I had to wait until every single person had left for the bike leg and then I was allowed access to my bike. It went downhill in a big way from there. It was hell; I was miles behind everyone else but I just wouldn't let myself quit. During the run they were packing up the drink stations as I went through!

When I got back to the finish line I was mortified to hear the claps and cheers, I just wanted to hide in a corner. To top it off my bike was the only bike left. They left a small section of the bike rack to hold up my bike and the rest was gone. I was so miserable it wasn't funny. I couldn't take any solace in the fact I had put myself through hell just so I could say I didn't quit.

On the way home in the car I started laughing, it really was laughable and I had Steve's famous last words ringing in my ears. I have yet to see Steve again but when I do I will be letting him know that this time round, that 'someone' was me!

As horrifyingly uncomfortable as that experience was, it reaffirmed for me that I was as tough as old boots and when push came to shove I knew I could back myself to finish the job.

It was ugly but I didn't quit when every single ounce of me wanted to.

In your life you no doubt have many examples of when you quit or didn't finish something and there is a good chance these are the experiences you pull out as a reference point when you set a new goal. You begin to remind yourself of all the times you failed. If you dig deep enough I am sure you can find an equal amount of experiences where you overcame, where you didn't quit, where you succeeded, where you won. Too often these are not the experiences we focus on, instead we focus on the times we failed, lost, didn't finish, etc.

So dump all of the information you have gathered to support your belief that you always quit or fail at everything and in its place start to compile a list of all of the things you did finish.

Set a timer for 10 minutes and do not stop writing until the buzzer beeps.

Fill that page with line after line of your successes.

When you don't think you have any more keep your pen moving anyway.

Once you are done read over your list; here is the information you need to remind you that you can do anything you put your mind to.

The trick though, is to put your mind there first.

Put your mind where you want your body to follow.

PERSEVERANCE

Perseverance is probably my second favourite principle.

In martial arts training perseverance is everything.

Can't get a kick the first time? You try again. Can't get it the second, third, fiftieth and five thousandth time? You try again.

The ONLY way to master excellence is to persevere through the discomfort of feeling awkward performing whatever technique you are attempting, to then feeling competent, to feeling skilled, to mastery (and believe me I have yet to feel I have mastered anything even after 22 years!).

Perseverance has taught me some of my biggest lessons both inside the dojang and outside of it. It has also brought me some of my greatest rewards.

Perseverance is the important bit between setting your goals and achieving them.

When you first set a goal you are in a positive mindset, energised by it and fully engaged in the belief you can achieve it.

Along the way stuff happens; usually stuff called LIFE.

This can be anything from another draining fight with your partner forcing you to think long and hard about your future, mounting financial stresses or trying to juggle everything that is demanded of you throughout the course of your day.

In this state the hurdles you would have easily jumped over in the initial goal-setting phase now seem mountainous. This is where life begins to intrude and distract us from the business of achieving our goals, and if we aren't careful this is where the wheels will fall off.

Looking at your goals every single morning before you get out of bed and every night before you go to sleep helps you keep your goals in the front of your mind and enables you to push through the tough days.

A goal you feel distanced from is not going to be compelling enough to give you the drive you need to push through (persevere) when challenges arise and the going gets tough.

I developed a habit that changed my whole approach to goals with some ridiculous (in a good way) results.

I set my alarm 30 minutes early each day so I have time to make myself a cuppa, head back to bed and spend time with my goals.

Each day I read my goals, remind myself that every day I am getting closer to them.

I check in and review what I have managed over the past days and question whether I need to step things up a bit or whether I'm on track.

Next I set my INTENTIONS for the day.

This will include the mindset I wish to have for the day along with the things I want to get done.

An example of this is below.

> *Today my intentions are:*
>
> *To be energised by and not overwhelmed by my workload.*
>
> *I will be inspired by my goals and work with passion, energy and focus .*
>
> *I will be in flow and I will shift truckloads of work effortlessly and efficiently.*
>
> *I will eat well and kick training butt.*
>
> *I will write one chapter of my book, edit three articles for the magazine and teach three inspirational classes.*

These intentions energise me from the get go and I can barely wait to get out of bed and hit the ground running.

It also ensures that every single day my goals are in focus and I do something every day to work towards them.

At night I do the following:

> *Pour myself a small glass of wine and toast the day.*
>
> *I write down all the things I want to pat myself on the back for and toast each one.*
>
> *I then write a list of everything I am grateful for.*
>
> *I read my goals and know that I have moved another day closer and again assess if I need to step things up tomorrow or if I'm satisfied with where things are at.*

I then put a mark next to each goal I made some progress towards that day – this is usually every one of them.

Spending this time with myself is sacred and important.

It is during these times I journal and let my thoughts flow.

This is where you can really get to know yourself intimately and check in with how you are showing up in the world. Check in to see if you are living your daily actions in line with your values and beliefs and pull yourself back on track before you stray too far.

When you know yourself well and can remain grounded in what is important and meaningful to you it eliminates a lot of stress.

Making decisions is easy because it either fits with your values and beliefs or it doesn't. It is either taking you closer to your goals or it isn't. This is what I base every single decision on.

Your journal can help you get clarity on these things.

Do this every day and how can you not reach the goals you so dearly want to achieve?

Perseverance is a state of mind even when we are calling on it for physical gain.

In a training session when you feel you have nothing left, it is your body that will quit first and here is when you need to call on your mind to push through.

Imagine you are doing stair sprint repeats and have hit the wall at set 20 when your goal was 30.

Every cell in your body wants to quit and you are now wishing you were the sort of person who could quit ☺

What gets you through and allows you to hang on for another 10 sets?

Obviously perseverance – but what allows you to persevere?

It is knowing that quitting is not in alignment with your value system and quitting will mean taking a step away from your goal instead of closer, which is the whole point of the training session.

You know that you won't be able to live with yourself comfortably for the rest of the day knowing you quit because of this, and so the motivation to get through is higher than the motivation to quit.

Once you make the decision not to quit you can get your head in the game and get the job done.

Some of you may be under the misconception that 'mentally tough' means you never have the desire to quit.

This could not be further from the truth.

The harder you push yourself, and the bigger the goal you are trying to achieve, trust me, the more you have times you want to quit!

Having the thoughts to quit doesn't make you weak, it makes you human.

It is what you do with and after the thought, that determines whether or not you wish to be ordinary or extraordinary.

Because you are human there will be times when you will quit and often these are the times we learn again just how important following through is for us. These times remind us of the consequences we suffer when we don't follow through.

There is always a lesson to help us become more of who we wish to be (are).

SELF-CONTROL

In Martial Arts Training it is during sparring where we need to exercise self-control the most and for good reason.

If you are out of control the feedback is immediate and brutal - lose it and you get smashed.

Lack of control allows your opponent to watch you unravel. It gives them a higher sense of calm and a sense of time standing still. It gives them the ability to pick off points and take joy from watching you self-combust. They know they have won.

A fighter not in control is ugly, and often previously learnt skills go right out the window.

If your own life being out of control is also ugly, isn't it?

When you are in control of the important things in your life everything flows and you experience calm and efficiency.

When out of control, even if it is in only one area of your life, you know about it.

You are in a constant state of anxiety, you always seem to be chasing your tail and never have enough time to do the things you need to get done or at least get them done properly.

There is no worse feeling than feeling out of control, feeling as though it doesn't matter what you try to do, you just can't seem to get it together.

In class I see this happen all the time.

A student will be having a particularly frustrating session where nothing seems to go right and they crack it. Not with anyone else but with themselves. You can see them sink further and further into frustration. You witness the wheels falling off anything they attempt from then on.

When I see this going on, I let them wrestle with it for a little while until they are almost puce with rage at themselves and then I step in.

I remind them that if they focus on the problem they will get more of it, whereas if they empty their mind and simply focus on the particular skill at hand, take the emotion out of it and only focus on fixing the technique, they will find themselves focusing on the solution instead of the problem.

Essentially I am asking them to summon up their inner white belt and to shed the noise going on in their heads and come at it with clarity. You can only do this without mental noise and tension in your body.

When you feel yourself losing or out of control, I ask you to do the same.

Channel your inner white belt and start with the simple. Start back at the basics.

Empty your mind of the noise and begin to focus on the solution.

I promise this turns it around every time!

HUMILITY

In martial arts there is always someone who can kick your butt and sometimes it will be the most unlikely candidate, especially if you let your ego run around unhindered.

For some black belt students there is nothing more humiliating than having a lower belt student kick them in the head.

If this happens it is usually because ego has entered the equation and the black belt has underestimated the lower-ranked student. In turn they are delivered a very fine lesson in humility ☺

Lessons in humility usually enter our lives when we need pulling into line because our egos have become unchecked. I'm not just talking in the dojang either.

I don't know about you, but for me recognising I've been a little too big for my boots is one of the most uncomfortable feelings in the world.

When you are shown clearly and suddenly that you are becoming a little too big for your boots it makes you want to say "OUCH!"

You know those times when you think you know everything (or is this just me??)

I have a girlfriend who I love dearly and who knows me pretty well.

I had been on a bit of a roll and things were falling into place for me personally and in business, and I was on top of the world. Happy to hand out advice to anyone who stood still for long enough.

This wasn't the problem though.

The problem was I couldn't take even the suggestion of advice from anyone else.

This certainly wasn't deliberate and I couldn't see for myself that I had been rejecting the friendly advice coming from my friends to "slow down" and "take it easy on yourself" when I was stressing out about a particularly challenging time, trying to fit everything into my week.

My dear friend then suggested she might get a T-shirt printed up for me with the words "I CAN'T BE TOLD" written across the front so people would know this up front and not even attempt to offer any advice.

WOW!! Was that not a smackdown lesson in humility right there?!

We laughed about it at the time and it was not meant in any way to be malicious, but I did go home and ponder this and try to look at it from the other person's view.

These people cared for me and knew me. They had their own wisdom and experience that I could greatly benefit from if I had just shut up and listened.

It was what I needed to remind me that I don't know everything and I should keep a more open mind.

I'm particularly guilty of this when it comes to listening to anyone in the fitness industry and if I look at a training or nutrition plan, I ALWAYS modify it my way because in my mind I know better. Actually this is probably a bad example because I'm not ready to give this thought up just yet!!

In your own life where is it you think you know better AND is it negatively affecting your progress?

There is a good chance this is showing up in the area you are struggling with the most and you don't even realize it.

Out of habit I reject advice before I've even heard it even if I smile and infer I'm taking it all in.

Sometimes it can be weeks before the conversation comes back to me and I take something from it.

This is a habit I am desperately trying to change.

Is there a habit you also need to change around this?

INTEGRITY

In my world of martial arts Integrity means four things:

1: Always behave with integrity around lower belt students; do not ever, ever use your higher ranking to intimidate or belittle a lower belt student in any way.

2: Mean what you say and say what you mean.

3: Be true to yourself, your values, and your word.

4: Live your life in accordance with what you know to be true and right for you.

Let me break these four rules of integrity down for you:

Always behave with integrity around lower belt students; do not ever, ever use your higher ranking to intimidate a lower belt in any way.

You may or may not ever learn a martial art (of course I hope you do!) and so you may not be exposed to lower belts in martial arts training, but you will be exposed to white belts in different areas of your life.

White belts in life can be people in your workplace with less experience or common sense; they can be the overweight person next to you on the treadmill at the gym; or they can be a family member who can't seem to get it together; and it is likely that on some level you judge them and behave towards them based on your own standards and experiences – something we all do.

In Martial Arts one of the best ways to learn is to teach, because the repetition of teaching the same thing over and over again helps ingrain the skill until it becomes automatic. It is also a wonderful reminder for the instructor to realize how far they have come themselves. Use the opportunity to share the lessons you have learned in life with the people around you who have yet to learn them for themselves. It helps you to reinforce the lesson for yourself, it often brings with it new insights and at the same time and aside from that it helps us to create a shift in our own thinking towards others.

Think for a moment of a white belt beginning martial arts at my dojang and my role as their instructor. I welcome the student first as a person and then as a student and a complete newcomer to my art. I see the person, understand their reason for wanting to begin and also do my best to uncover how much courage it took them to walk through the door. In the extreme what happens next can go either one of two ways: The beginner is a quick and respectful learner and is both easy and a pleasure to teach, or, they are a nightmare in either or both attitude and ability.

In my early days as an instructor I dreaded the latter and while I hope they never caught on I wished like heck they would go and find something else to do, because it did my head in explaining a technique in great detail only to have them produce a technique that looked nothing like what I had shown them. My judgment was high and I just could not understand how someone could get it so wrong and I knew it was not as a result of my efforts!

In my early years of training I often judged people based on their ability and I can clearly remember asking my instructor one day, "How can that guy be a black belt when he can't even kick past his waist? He is terrible." Sadly I was slow on the uptake and asked this question more than once. Each time my instructor would say, "Not everyone has your physical ability and being a black belt is not all about your physical skills, it is also about your commitment and love of the martial art and what you bring to the club and your fellow students." It took me a while to get my head around this because in my arrogance I figured if you are a black belt you have to be able to kick butt.

Over the years my instructor pointed out a number of black belts who I thought were sadly lacking and he shared their stories with me. I then began to understand that, for example, the lady with the black hair had overcome cancer more than once and she was there for her mental health and the support of her fellow students. The old man in his 80s who never kicked but turned up week after week, had also earned his right to be there.

When I opened my own school an older male student who had a very disfigured spine and a number of other health-related issues began training with me. Now as a 44-year-old woman, I can finally appreciate just how courageous he was to be training alongside younger and fitter, more able-bodied students. I was a hard taskmaster and don't think I gave him much latitude. He was expected to perform at the best of his ability and in fact he rarely missed a class and was always so happy to be training despite how hard it was for him physically. I only hope that as a woman in my 20s I showed him the respect I now know he so rightly deserved.

Thankfully over the years I have learnt some humility and developed a deep sense of respect for everyone who passes through my dojang door, because I now know how hard it is for some people just to make that very first step.

However, one thing has never changed and that is my assertion that every single student, regardless of age, shape, size, ability or anything else, MUST work to the best of THEIR ability. I now completely understand (especially as I get older!) that not everyone's body is capable of the same things, but every person is capable of doing their best.

The best way you can honour yourself is to have the highest integrity in your dealings with the people around you. You are never going to love everyone you come across in your life, but try your best to understand what makes a person tick and allow for your differences. To know you are a good person in the way you treat and interact with others is priceless and will bring with it a very deep sense of fulfilment.

Mean what you say and say what you mean – a matter of trust.

Imagine for a moment that you come along to my Taekwondo class as a beginner student and you tell me you are worried about contact sparring. I tell you that as a beginner you do not need to be concerned with contact sparring in the first one to three months of your training (depending on your specific progress). In your mind this brings with it a huge amount of relief and frees your mind to be able to focus on enjoying your training and improving.

Then imagine if two weeks after you have paid your money I tell you to put on a body shield for sparring and being a beginner you are too intimidated to say you are not ready.

This would be a gross breach of trust between student and instructor and the likelihood of the student ever trusting another thing I say (if they even stay) is highly unlikely. Once trust like that is broken it is very hard to rebuild. This is especially true if the issue is a hot one for the student.

How does this relate?

Have you ever promised your best friend, a member of your family or your partner that today was the day and that things were going to change around here?

Did you tell them that things would be different and that you were not going to stop until you reached your goal?

And then didn't?

Have you done it more than once?

More than 10 times?

Is it also true that you have become completely frustrated with this person when they don't get giddy with excitement and have unwavering belief in you this time round?

Deep down you know that the frustration is really with yourself and not the other party, because it just reminds you that you didn't follow through all of the other times and they quite rightly don't believe a word you say with respect to you reaching your goal.

This is some of the mental clutter I'm talking about, taking up space and making you feel miserable about yourself.

You can knock that on the head by only saying what you mean and meaning what you say. Before you go ahead and make any more grand announcements, stop and think if you really, truly mean what you are about to say, and if you do, you must act on it until it is fulfilled.

Write down the things you have promised to those closest to you over and over again.

Which items are still relevant and which ones are still floating around simply because you haven't taken the time to re-evaluate and discard because they are no longer a priority?

What are the items you deep down know you have to fulfil because if you don't, you know they will haunt you forever?

Put them in order of priority and set them aside for later.

Be true to yourself, your values, and your word.

In my opinion there is no greater freedom from internal struggle than when you live true to yourself, your values and your word.

Think about it for a moment.

How do you feel when you are not living true to yourself and your values and not honouring your word? It feels rotten. It causes massive amounts of stress and often self-loathing. Bundle all of that up together and life is certainly no longer a party! Before you know it you are grumpy with the world, your productivity suffers, as does your health and your relationships. You are not fun to be around and you know it, so you start to withdraw from the human race. This can last a few days or a few years, but it happens.

It happens because it weighs heavily on you and pulls you downwards. We all have values, whether we have spent time discovering our unique values or not, they are there. If we are not living in alignment with them it begins to cause us problems in the form of more mental clutter and noise that then goes on to manifest itself in the things I talked about above.

An enlightening lesson in values and being true to myself came to me in the form of being asked to cast for a popular TV reality show that did not fit my values for even a second. By casting I would essentially be saying to myself, "I am prepared to put aside everything I know to be true and ethical for the sake of building my media profile." The decision was very easy for me. It was a no-brainer because I knew I could not live outside my values comfortably and I know myself well enough to know everything around and within me would suffer and there was no way I was willing to go there simply for the sake of a media profile.

Interestingly, not long after that other opportunities showed up (not in TV) that very strongly resonated with my values. I see that as my reward for staying true and honest to my values and word.

Being true to your word does not in any way need to be about the big stuff, in fact being true to your word consistently on a daily basis is where the true power of it is realized, especially in relation to the thing you struggle with most.

For example if your biggest struggle is your relationship with food (and it is for sooo many women), then by simply honouring your word not to eat crap or starve yourself will bring you much peace and pride. You know how the opposite feels when every day you tell yourself you will only eat healthy food and avoid the foods you know you shouldn't be eating day in day out. You give your word to yourself and then you break it and it feels like shite! It triggers emotions of failure and self-loathing and so the spiral begins again until you once again give your word to yourself you will only eat healthy food and avoid junk. It is a vicious cycle.

Every time you break your word to yourself you reinforce the belief you are useless (or whatever this word is for you). Again this creates mental clutter and noise filling your head and contributing to the overwhelm. This is not where you want to live!

In contrast, every time you make a promise to yourself and keep it, you grow a little stronger and a little prouder and the belief that you can do this slowly grows. The more you honour your word to yourself, the stronger this becomes.

It seems like such a simple thing and yet it can be one of the hardest things to master. Often the reason it is so hard to master is because we give it more power than it actually has. We create a 'thing' around it that often sounds something like this: "I am an emotional eater and I have no control", when this is simply not the case. You do have control; in fact you are the ONLY one in control, I mean who else is there? By handing control over to an imaginary power you then feel powerless to resist, when in reality you control the shots, every single one of them.

When you hand over power it is a way to give yourself permission to continue down this path; "it's not my fault, I'm an emotional eater". This says you are powerless and you know you are not. You simply need to get into the practice of honouring your word to yourself. At times it will be difficult and this is the reason it is easier to hand over power, so you don't have to face the difficult part and work through it. But you can. The only alternative is to continue the way you are and live with the consequences. The fact you are reading this tells me you do want to change and you wish to avoid those consequences. I know you can do it and it all starts by honouring your word (to yourself).

A woman's relationship with food is the obvious one to choose, because I know through my online businesses and the women I work with day in day out that so many woman struggle with this on a daily basis . For you it may not be food but regardless the lessons are the same. The exercise below will help you develop some more clarity around this.

What are the promises you make to yourself that you routinely break? (Write them all down, have a brain dump and get it all out.)

How does it make you feel every time you let yourself down by breaking your word?

What are the consequences of continually breaking your word?

What will happen if you continue on this path?

How would you like it to be?

Live your life in accordance with what you know to be true and right for you.

You may be thinking that these are all variations of the same theme and you are probably right, but I also know that repetition is the mother of skill and if I harp on about it long enough you won't be able to ignore it!

Just like honouring your word, living in accordance with what you know to be true and right for you will help unshackle you from the mental clutter and noise, because the internal battle ceases when you do so.

We all have a different truth and what is right for one person is often not for another. Here we need to stand strong and find out what our individual beliefs and values are so we can live in accordance with them.

This is why kids often get into so much trouble – peer group pressure – usually because they are yet to form solid foundations for themselves and so they can be easily influenced by those around them. This is not to say they don't have an inner compass, they are just not yet ready to follow it, because it is not as important to them as being one of the crowd.

As adults, by now we should have fully grasped what we know to be right for us and true to our values and beliefs, and it is up to us to have the strength and courage to live by this.

I know women who train hard and eat well and I think they are doing great, only to discover they smoke cigarettes! On a deep level these women know that they highly value being healthy, fit and lean, so this just doesn't fit at all and they know smoking isn't right despite kidding themselves that they make up for it in other ways.

I know this one first hand because when I started Taekwondo I was a smoker, I actually still can't quite believe I ever did it!

I grew up in a family where everyone smoked; my grandparents on both sides, my uncles and aunties, and my parents. It seemed like a right of passage, just something you did.

But there was always a niggling in my gut telling me I shouldn't be doing it. Once I started training my instructor pointed out that smoking and Taekwondo didn't go hand in hand. I was working weekends in a pub so giving up was going to be hard, especially at knock-off drinks time.

When I saw the reactions of some of the people I trained with when they discovered I smoked, I also had to face that what my gut was telling me was right. This was not the right thing for me to be doing. I set myself a date one month ahead and promised myself I would quit on that day, and I did!

In that month I troubleshooted all of the situations I would encounter that would be hard to handle and I came up with an action plan.

I was so excited I wanted to give up there and then, but I made myself keep smoking till D Day – so in the end it was: "Oh God, do I have to smoke again??!!"

I found that all of the work I had done ahead of time helped me a lot, because when I faced the situations I dreaded it was like I had already been there and I just rolled out my plan of action.

I can't tell you the relief I felt from giving up; in the early days I would often dream I had smoked again and I would wake up in such a panic because I wasn't a smoker anymore and I was repulsed by the thought of it.

The relief came from living what I knew to be right for me, and smoking wasn't it. You probably have your own version of this; it could be drinking too much, not exercising, watching mind-numbing TV, not spending enough time with your kids, not apologizing to someone you know you should, etc.

Your gut will tell you what is right and true for you so practice listening to what it is telling you and be guided by it.

Where are you living outside your values?

How are you going to change this TODAY?

COURAGE

It took me a while to realize that courage is not the absence of fear but acting in the face of that fear.

I always thought that all of the nerves and anxiety I had in the lead up to a fight meant I was weak and I certainly didn't feel courageous. It took a very close and extremely tough Martial Arts friend of mine telling me he always felt that way before a fight for me to understand that this was normal. He also pointed out that the courage was in stepping in to the ring in the first place, along with all of the sparring that got me ready to step onto the mat.

Looking from the outside in it's true and I have the utmost respect for anyone who has the courage to step on to the mat ready to do battle.

Obviously courage isn't all about fighting and you can build your courage muscle without ever having to step into the ring, but for me fighting has always been a reference point I fall back to.

The courage to change, the courage to stand by your convictions, the courage to challenge yourself and the courage to make another attempt at your goal are what I want to focus on in this section.

I want you to know, just as I had to learn, that feeling fear does not make you a coward, it simply means that the thing you are about to attempt or change means something to you, in fact it probably means mountains. If it didn't then you would not have the fear of failure hanging over your head. It is like that fabulous question: "What would you do if you knew you couldn't fail?"

Fear holds us back from really going for it in life so we must learn how to recognise it as fear, then uncover the root of the fear so we can address this and face it head on.

I'm the kind of girl who rips a Band-Aid off in one go, no stuffing about trying to make the process easier, if it has to come off then let's get the damn thing off. This is also my metaphor for life. I cannot wait for things to happen. I have to make them happen and if that means getting down and dirty with my fear so I can get past it, that's what I do. This is what I encourage you to do also. It's there, it is not going away so you might as well just get on with it.

We all know people who are waiting for things to happen for them or to come to them, when you and I both know that if they just went out and found it or got it done then the whole thing would be over with.

Stepping outside of your comfort zone takes courage, but personal growth and deep satisfaction often reside outside the comfort zone. I've never met anyone who achieved anything great in their life, who didn't have to scare themselves silly to get there.

This is what it takes.

Have you been putting off signing up for your first Martial Arts Class or 5kms fun run or first Marathon or first gym membership? Does the thought of stepping outside your comfort zone scare the crap out of you? If it does that is AWESOME, because it means big stuff will happen for you once you take that first step. If it scares you it is worth doing, if it scares you it means you have probably been battling this internal battle for a long time and let me tell you now, that battle isn't going anywhere until you quiet the beast and you can only quite the beast by signing your name on the dotted line and doing it.

Maybe your fear is committing fully to change; sometimes it goes like this...

I really want to change my body and get fit... but I'm not a runner so I'm not going to run.

OR

I really want to lose weight... but I'm not willing to give up my wine.

OR

I really want to join the gym and start training everyday... but I really don't like the way the other people in the gym look at me because I am overweight.

What you need to do is go with the first part of the sentence (whatever it is for you) and discard the rest, the part that comes after "but".

If you have the thought in the first place it means the seed is planted and unless you go for it, it will be like a bug up your butt until you do it.

I have women who train at my dojang who are experiencing being as fit as an athlete and looking and feeling fabulous for the first time EVER in their 30s and 40s and the common theme amongst them all is that they wished they had started training a decade or more ago.

Don't fall into the trap of telling yourself you will do this "when"... when the kids are at school, when you are fitter, when your friend can come with you. All of these things are just resistance that is coming from your fear, nothing more and nothing less.

When you feel the resistance, either in the form of excuses or genuine fear, pick it apart and give it some perspective.

What is the worst thing that can happen if you take up Martial Arts?

You could be in the best shape of your life, you could learn to defend yourself and the people dear to you, you could start living the type of lifestyle that sees you fit and healthy for the rest of your life and be a role model to those you love.

What is the best thing that could happen if you take up Martial Arts?

Hmm… the list looks pretty much the same!!

Seriously though, go through the process of what is the worst thing that could happen. For me it was coming last in the triathlon… and it happened but no-one died. The worst happened and no-one died. I got over it and I also received another lesson in humility (my martial arts principle nemesis). Keep it in perspective and spend A LOT of time thinking about the best things that can happen from making the change or signing up and settle the fear, so you can get on with going for it.

In Taekwondo, courage is called upon often and takes on many forms and degrees depending on the circumstances.

Whenever you strap on your sparring gear, walk on to the mat and face up against a competitive opponent, courage is required.

When you step on the mat in competition, much greater courage is required.

Courage is required for every colour belt grading and bucket loads more is needed for black belt gradings.

For some it takes a mountain of courage just to walk through the door.

Courage and fear usually go hand in hand.

Here is a good time to remember that courage is not the absence of fear, but forcing yourself to move forward in spite of the fear.

The fear makes it an even greater achievement in the end.

Fear is what keeps us sharp and overcoming fear makes the reward even greater; however the fear is not what we want to be focused on.

Courage and fear go hand in hand, but so do courage and confidence, and confidence can help us overcome fear. So what we want to focus on is getting ourselves to a place of confidence so we are prepared to act.

If we use the example of a full contact sparring competition it would make a lot of sense NOT to enter the event if you are having your butt kicked in every training session and lack confidence; you just wouldn't do it.

What leads a competitor to the mat is often not 100% confidence, but enough confidence to garner the courage needed to take the leap.

This confidence comes from climbing a mountain and that mountain is becoming fight ready and all that that means: months of gruelling training and often dieting. Somewhere in amongst the training things start to come together, you feel more comfortable with your sparring, you experience some wins and from here your confidence grows and this gives you the courage to step onto the mat.

Again outside of the dojang we can use the example of tackling the task of losing a large amount of weight and getting yourself fit and healthy.

If you have experienced many past failures it would not be unusual to feel gun-shy and doubt your ability to follow through and achieve.

Your confidence may be at an all-time low and it can be very hard to start when feeling this way. This is where courage is required just to begin.

Courage doesn't need to be big; sometimes courage is quiet, as in this case.

It is in the moment we decide to try again we step into our courage, but the job is not done yet and often the first bang of courage can turn into the fizzle of another aborted attempt.

In this moment of courage we need to begin to build confidence and we do this by setting ourselves up to win small and often.

The more wins, the greater confidence grows, and with greater confidence comes greater reserves of courage we can tap into to aim higher.

There are many opportunities to test your courage and looking for these opportunities and testing yourself is a good habit to get into.

I like to test my courage in some way every single day; feeling courageous makes me feel strong and reminds me that there is always more, there is always another level.

The ways I test myself are not always big, it can be as simple as sharing an opinion on Facebook or pumping the treadmill up to a speed I haven't been able to manage before.

The trick is to grab the opportunity when it's there and just go with it.

If I'm on the treadmill and feeling good then that is the time to attempt it right there and then.

If I go away and think about it and plan for it next time maybe I'll overthink it and stress over it and talk myself out of it before I even start. I'll put it off and off until I give up on it so I'm not going to take that chance, if the opportunity shows up I'm on it.

Too often we wait until we are 'ready', till the time is 'perfect' to start, but the truth is there is no perfect time, there is just time and so there is little point in waiting for that.

You have shown great courage in your life already and now is the time to reflect on this.

Think about the times in your life when you have been fearful of something but done it anyway, the examples don't have to be big but I'll bet you have some big ones in there too.

Start a list and keep writing for 15 minutes. Do not stop until the clock hits 15 then look back over the list and ask yourself how you feel?

EXCELLENCE

Ahhh… excellence.

Just seeing the word in writing makes me aspire to it.

It is the bar above all others and it is the one I happily set for myself and those around me.

This is what separates the wheat from the chaff.

Recently I interviewed our Sydney 2000 Gold Medallist, Lauren Burns, for my magazine (you can get download the audio and see the article at BlackBeltWomanMag.com).

Lauren is a true champion; I had the honour of training alongside her on State team and watched her fight many times.

In her interview she said some simple words that inspired much excitement and sense of possibility for me.

The mentioned that her coach drummed into them to… here it is …

To do the simple things with excellence.

Right away my mind went to all of the things I was rushing through in my life that could be improved upon profoundly if I just took the time for excellence in the simple things.

I also knew the impact this would have on the bigger stuff.

I knew that excellence in the simple and small things in life would ensure I slowed down and paid attention.

So I want you to start there; seeking excellence in even the smallest most mundane of tasks and noticing how your mind changes.

Since hearing those magical words I find I am doing less in each day but unlike in the past, I don't feel the need to go back and check and recheck because I wasn't 100% happy with it the first time on account of rushing it.

I have always held excellence high on my list of values so I was interested to see that while I embraced it in its larger context I was missing it in the detail.

You know you are not seeking excellence when you find yourself saying, "This is good enough" or "This will do for now."

Excellence isn't delivered through good enough; it comes from taking the time to do the small and the simple with excellence.

All these little examples of excellence add up to become excellence in all areas of your life.

Where are you taking short cuts?

Where would practicing excellence in the small and simple have the greatest impact in your life?

PART THREE:

TRAINING YOUR WAY TO A KICKASS BODY

If you are not already training in Martial Arts, I highly recommend you go and try out a few different clubs in your area and just give it a go.

You have nothing to lose by giving it a try and if you are lucky you will find a club and an instructor that lights the fire in your belly.

That said you can train like a Martial Artist for the fitness benefits without ever setting foot in a dojang.

My style of Taekwondo is 95% kicking.

Because we use the largest muscle groups in our bodies to kick (core/legs/glutes) we burn a ton of calories.

For women kicking styles do much more than just burn a ridiculous amount of calories, they also strengthen and tone the lower body like nothing else.

If you have struggled to gain a six pack, tight tooshie and killer thighs then look no further than Taekwondo.

Because of the intensity of the training in Marital Arts it truly does transform your body and your mind like nothing else. (You simply cannot train at intensity without the mind entering the equation.)

Over the years I have dipped my toe in a few other pursuits (all the while continuing with my Taekwondo training) and only then did I realize how much my martial arts training had assisted my body and mind.

I have had many students over the years who come to me already at a high standard of fitness, only to be shocked at how physically demanding Taekwondo training is. But at the same time they also say that they don't realize how hard they are working because they are thinking so much.

Unless I am what I deem "Fight Fit" I don't feel fit at all.

To feel Fight Fit I need all of the following boxes to be ticked:

1:   I can sprint repeatedly both on the flat and on stairs or hills.

2:   I can do plyometrics till the cows come home.

3:   I'm fast and my reaction speed is good.

4:   I feel strong but light and fast.

5:    My timing and rhythm are sharp.

6:    I have the ability to absorb and deliver impact repeatedly.

7:    I feel flexible and loose.

8:    I'm ALWAYS sore!!

Who doesn't want to feel fight fit and reap the benefits of the type of training that gives you all of the above, regardless of whether or not you ever step onto the mat to fight?

I had taken for granted how fit I was when I was competing because I never ever felt fit. Years later as I began to train my own fighters I realized this was simply because I was always pushing the envelope of my physical ability and because of this training was never, ever easy or comfortable. Looking back I can now see just how ridiculously fit I was.

One example of not feeling fit back then was our warm-up run; we used to run a 3km route after doing stair work and I thought I was hopeless at it, because it was so hard and nearly killed me every single time.

We were running a little over 3km in around 9 minutes – now I get why it was hard, but back then I had no running reference points to realize this was a cracking pace and that this is why it was so bloody hard!

These days I have times when my fitness is close or equal to that and thankfully with the added years I can get my mind where it needs to be to perform and push through a tough session much faster and more easily than what I could do in my 20s.

These days I can also recognize when I'm in peak shape based on my now many years of experience.

I have run half marathons and I trained for the Paris Marathon (I did this for my 40th). Unfortunately I went to Paris injured and didn't finish. In fact I only ran 30k which was less distance than I had run in my training runs.

Distance running kicks my butt and to be honest I found that I never felt LESS fit than when I trained for a Marathon. Here I was expecting to sacrifice some speed and fast twitch, but I never expected to feel so unfit when I could run 35kms!! Who knew, right??

What it came down to was that my body is used to going hard for short explosive bursts, followed by short recovery phases and when I train like that I feel freaking awesome.

I feel fast and sharp and strong and it gives me a wonderful base to build from so that if I do want to do a short distance triathlon or run a 10 or 15 or 21kms, I know I am starting from a good, strong base and I can take the direction of my training in any way that I choose and be ready to go.

Training in Martial Arts doesn't mean you can't do anything else and in fact cross training can make you a better all-round athlete. However, you do need to be mindful of what your training priority is at that particular time, so you are not doing two types of training that fight against each other, as I did when I was training simultaneously for a marathon (endurance) and Taekwondo training (explosive speed and power).

When you are training in Martial Arts you need to train for a number of things and all of these things add up to feeling fight fit.

Explosive Speed

Power

Agility

Flexibility

Reaction

Balance and co-ordination.

And you need to be able to repeat all of these things over and over again.

Importantly, we also need some endurance for numerous bouts of three rounds. Over the course of a competition day you need to be able to back up fight after fight after fight, unlike boxing where you have one bout, we can have any number of fights depending on how many participants are entered into that particular weight division; three, four and five fights aren't unusual on competition day.

There are so many facets to Taekwondo training, which is why I love it so, so much. You will benefit from Martial Arts training whether or not you train at home or at your local dojang.

The other thing I love about Taekwondo training is that the training can be modified.

All types of bodies and all ages can train for different purposes and for different phases of training life.

I trained through both my pregnancies and in fact was training on both the days I gave birth to my children.

Training can be modified for injuries and interests as well.

You may not be able to contact spar due to an impact injury, but you can still fresh air kick.

You may not love contact sparring, but love kicking pads and bags and perfecting your patterns.

There is always some purpose to be found in training.

Martial Arts training is not like a fitness class where all you are getting from it is fitness and perhaps some stress release. There is always so much more to gain.

It can be easy to want to ditch training because you can't kick or punch or throw due to injury when this is your favourite part of the class. Being a true martial artist, embracing discipline and commitment, the right thing to do is turn up at every class regardless, find an angle you can work and go home glad you did.

As I mentioned earlier there are many facets to Taekwondo training and to feeling fight fit.

And so now we get to the fun part and start talking training!

With so many facets coming into play it can be tempting to want to tackle them all at once and if you are anything like me then you want to go hell for leather and tackle them all at once and tackle them all hard.

Trust me, this always ends in disaster and I'm speaking from first-hand experience. It seems to be my destiny to find out things the hard way!

Overtraining symptoms, injury and burnout are on the cards if you take this approach and what you end up with is a lot of time on the sidelines.

It is much better to take a progressive approach, taking care to tackle each facet in its rightful place, and build on your progress over time letting your body adapt and then with a strong base, you can ramp it up.

There is a right way and a wrong way to go from 0 to 100 and I am pretty sure I have come close to unearthing all of them! By forcing my body to perform higher level skill tasks before disciplining myself to work through the lower level stuff, I repeatedly came unstuck and ended up on the sidelines.

A good example of this is not Taekwondo related but running related.

I have had a spate of lower leg and hip issues that meant I spent a lot of time at the physio. It did not matter how many times my wonderful (and patient, the man deserves a medal!!) physio insisted that if I could not hop at least 15 times on my dodgy leg (hip, ankle, calf knee – take your pick) I shouldn't be running. But, I didn't listen.

So here I was with a bad calf tear thinking as the pain wasn't 'that bad' that I could run. So run I did, and it was ugly: having to land on my heel (when I am a mid-foot striker) and not being able to push off the ball of my foot.

The result?

An even worse tear within three weeks that sidelined me for 16 weeks instead of the original –four to five.

So the moral of that story is… don't try to run before you can hop!

And the take away is not to force your body to perform higher level tasks if you haven't put in the work on the lower level tasks (this includes rehab) because it almost always ends in tears.

And for all you stubborn ones, (like me) here are some words that changed my thinking – just because you **"can"** doesn't mean you **"should"**.

Because my body could push through a plyometric session without first having done standard strength then power work I would do it… again and again and again (and end up injured). So now when I'm about to do something dumb I ask myself, "You know you can do this, but should you be doing it?", and this forces me to look at the bigger picture; do I really want to risk injury and time on the sidelines for the sake of one awesome training session… (hmmm… let's try that again) one training session at a higher intensity than my body can sustain at the time.

So now we know there is (or should be) a natural order to things let's talk about what that looks like when you're starting with an absolute beginner.

AEROBIC BASE

Pretty quickly we want to be doing sprint work because it perfectly complements martial arts training, gets you in great shape and burns a ton of calories. But before we get to that we need a good aerobic base which, in my opinion, is the boring but absolutely necessary bit and something I always avoided, which meant my endurance always suffered.

A good aerobic base means our muscles are trained to keep a supply of oxygen when training at a lower intensity over time. Lower intensity training allows our body enough time to supply the muscles with oxygen and oxygen fuels your muscles, keeping you moving for an unlimited amount of time if we remain at the right intensity.

In our training we don't want to be running any marathons, but we want to be able to crank out an easy 5kms without too much of an effort.

A good aerobic base also means we recover better from the higher intensity stuff and we just feel 'better' or more comfortable in our training.

We don't want to give a lot of time to aerobic conditioning once we have our base, and one or two 30-40 minute runs a week is enough once that base is established.

In this phase our bodies are predominantly utilizing the basic aerobic system and this is where we build our base.

What this does is set us up to be able to safely add speed work where we begin to predominantly train our anaerobic system using both Lactic Acid and ATP-PC anaerobic systems (more on this soon).

ANAEROBIC TRAINING

The anaerobic system is where energy is produced in the absence of oxygen, which then creates the by-product: lactic acid. Lactic acid is what makes our legs 'tired' and heavy and we feel as though we are about done.

It is also the build-up of lactic acid that gives us the feeling of nausea and sometimes vomiting (if you're lucky ☺).

The Lactic Acid System is used at the start of exercise (in the first few minutes), as the body cannot yet deliver oxygen to the muscles fast enough to initiate the chemical reactions which occur during aerobic metabolism. It is also used as we increase our intensity and our aerobic system can no longer keep up the delivery of enough oxygen rich blood to the muscles.

We are training under the Lactic Acid System when we do longer running speed repeats or bag work of up to around two minutes.

Training our Lactic Acid System (sometimes also simply referred to as the anaerobic system) means we can train to hold off fatigue; the longer we can hold off fatigue the better, because this means we can train more comfortably for longer periods and we all want that, right?

Once we have reached sufficient conditioning in these two systems we can then begin to challenge our bodies further and train our ATP-CP System and this is where we get to sprint (finally!!).

ATP (Adenosine Triphosphate) is a high-energy molecule broken down to form ADP (Adenosine Diphosphate) and release energy. PC (Phosphocreatine) is another high-energy molecule found in the Sarcoplasm of the muscle fibres.

The breakdown of ATP and the increase of ADP triggers the enzyme Creatine Kinase to initiate the breakdown of PC into phosphate and creatine, and this provides the energy required to resynthesise APT at a rapid rate. If you find this a little too confusing, don't worry, it's not necessary to understand the science.

As we only have 120g of creatine in our bodies at any time, the repeated breakdown of PC and resynthesis of ATP is only temporary and can only last for around 10 seconds.

We are training our ATP-CP system when we do a flat out sprint of around 10 seconds.

As explained earlier, when we work in the Anaerobic System (lactic acid or ATP-PC) our muscles are working in the absence of oxygen. Once you have completed your effort, your muscles are in what we call "Oxygen Debt".

Oxygen debt means your respiration rate will be very high (you are huffing and puffing like nobody's business) as your body works to return oxygen to the muscles.

This can be confused with being unfit, but this is simply not the case.

If you watch a 100m sprint or 50m freestyle event at the Olympics you see athletes huffing and puffing like crazy for ages afterwards, even if their event only lasts 10 seconds.

This is certainly not because they are unfit, but simply because their muscles are in oxygen debt and trying to recover.

The more conditioned you become the better conditioned your body becomes at returning the oxygen to the muscles, so recovery is always a really great way to gauge progress, in fact this is my preferred method for gauging improved fitness in my students.

Through the type of training we have undertaken to develop our aerobic base and then our blood lactate (or anaerobic / lactic acid) threshold, we have now conditioned our bodies to be able to cope with higher level, more demanding skills, because our muscles and tendons are now strong enough to cope with increased intensity.

Imagine coming off the couch after an extended time being sedentary and your first training session involves a flat out sprint for 10 seconds up a steep hill.

That has tendon tears written all over it, because the body is just not ready to cope with those demands.

You should only be training hard sprint work when you have done the work building your body up to this. I promise you not only will you be more comfortable performing at this level, but it will also mean much less chance of injury.

In summary it looks like this:

> 1: Build aerobic base for four weeks (give or take, depending on the individual) by doing low intensity, steady state aerobic conditioning.
>
> 2: Train Lactic Acid System for four weeks (again give or take) by adding some speed work and building on your progress each week, i.e., start with 1 min at 3km pace and each week increase time at the same pace until you hit the 2 minute mark and then work on improving speed.
>
> 3: Introduce ATP-CP System – You won't let go of your low intensity sessions or your speed work, but you will now add 1-3 (you know the drill by now) explosive sprint sessions each week. You can even combine your aerobic sessions with these and add the sprints at the end.

Training in this manner not only takes care of your cardiovascular fitness, but it also works your strength, power, speed and muscular endurance.

RESISTANCE TRAINING

To support all of this and to make our bodies even stronger, faster and more powerful (and injury resistant) we need to add resistance training for strength, power and speed and this means 'weights', ladies.

Again there is a natural order to things.

If strength is the amount of force that can be generated by a muscle when it is contracting, and power is the ability to combine strength with speed (to perform the contraction at speed), then it makes sense to train strength before power, does it not?

Trying to lift heavy resistance at speed before your body has had the chance to adapt to lifting resistance (heavy or not) is another recipe for disaster.

Strength is the lower level skill to power, just as the aerobic system is a lower skill level to ATP-PC.

When we lift weights we are putting our muscles under stress.

As we work the muscles with weights the individual muscle fibres tear and then repair themselves over the next 24 hours and this is how they become stronger and how we develop strength.

When we begin strength training we should start at a weight that is comfortable and allows us to maintain perfect form. Maintaining form is important to avoid injury and to develop the muscle correctly.

Within a short amount of time your muscles will have grown stronger and you will find you need to increase your weights because the ones you started with are now too light.

You don't need to change anything at this stage other than the amount of weight you are lifting.

Once you have been lifting and adding weight for a little while and have gained some good strength you can begin to safely start to add speed (explosive movement).

Initially you would drop your weights back while you added the extra stress of speed and work back up to the weight you were lifting before and then beyond.

Plyometric training can then be added, as this improves both strength and power.

In summary it looks like this:

1: Start with strength training at a comfortable weight with perfect form and work on increasing your weights (maintaining perfect form) until you have developed a good strength base – around four to eight weeks.

2: Introduce power by initially dropping the weights back and doing the movement with speed.

3: Introduce Plyometric Training.

Of course our cardiovascular and strength training are here as support to our Martial Arts training, giving us good fitness and a strong body able to cope with the demands of our martial arts training.

Here is where we begin to work on the specifics of our martial art.

MARTIAL ARTS SPECIFIC TRAINING

You can be as fast as the wind in sprint training, but if your timing and/or footwork skills are poor on the mat, it is of no use to your Martial Art and so this is where we begin to look at martial arts specific training.

Outside the classroom you can work the progression as we did with cardio and resistance.

For example you can start with 1 minute rounds on the bag and work up to 3 minutes over time. Then once you have 3 minute rounds nailed, you can increase the time or increase the power of your kicks or add more dynamic kicks or work on your speed to keep improving.

In class it is a different story because instructors like to throw students in at the deep end sometimes (or is this just me??) to force some growth.

This means you have to be ready for anything and sometimes you will be forced to work above your skillset. This is why all of the other training outside of the dojang is so important.

All of that other training keeps you fight fit and puts you in a great position to cope with anything your instructor throws at you.

You might still have your butt kicked by a faster or more experienced student because your Martial Art specific skills aren't yet as polished, but you will be fit and strong and be able to hold your own on all other levels.

Here are some examples of how we work to improve our Martial Arts specific skills.

Explosive Speed: Attack and counter drills with and without resistance bands.

Power: (this is trained outside the dojang with weights)

Balance/Agility: Footwork drills, Line Drills, kicking combinations designed to test agility.

Flexibility: Stretching, mostly dynamic but some passive

Timing/Reaction : Paddle reaction drills, timing drills on protectors.

You can see how stepping onto the mat with a strong, fit, agile and flexible body will help you to carry out all of this training more effectively.

All of that said, if you haven't started training in Martial Arts yet, not having this should not be a deterrent.

As a beginner your body will not be challenged in any major way for quite some time, as you are learning new skills and the majority of your time is spent working at a lower level as you work to perfect these.

The more you train the more skills you acquire and you will know when it is time to step things up outside the dojang, although I would recommend adding additional training outside the dojang as soon as you can.

As far as I'm concerned you can never be too fit or too strong or too prepared.

PULLING IT ALL TOGETHER

I know this is a lot of information to absorb so I'll break the training phases down into an easy sequence for you to follow.

1: BASE FITNESS and STRENGTH (let's say for the sake of argument six weeks)

3 – 5 / 20-40 minute Aerobic Base Building Cardio Sessions

I recommend running and cycling.

2- 4 / 40 minute Strength Sessions

I recommend doing a full body workout twice a week or a split program three to four times a week, whereby we break our workouts up into different body parts to be worked over different days of the week; for example, a simple two days split would be working upper body one day and lower body the next, a couple of rest days, then repeat – giving you four sessions over the course of the week.

2- 4 Classes or Skill Specific Training Sessions

If you are a beginner start with the minimum and work up.

2: INTRODUCING POWER AND LACTIC ACID SYSTEM TRAINING (four weeks)

Keep 1 x 20-40 minute Aerobic Base Building Cardio Sessions

Add 2 x 20-30 minute Lactic Acid Sessions

I recommend running speed sessions on the flat and on hills or stationary bike hills or speed work.

Start with 1 minute effort followed by 30sec to 1min recovery and each week add 30sec to 1min to the work phase.

Increase your speed where you can as well.

Drop your weights back on the strength exercises specific to your martial art and add explosive movement in the lift phase.

For example, for kicking styles squats and power lifts are ideally performed at speed.

2- 4 Classes or Skill Specific Training Sessions

3: INTRODUCING PLYOs and ATP-PC SYSTEM TRAINING (four weeks)

Keep 1 x 20-40 minute Aerobic Base Building Cardio Sessions

Keep 1 x 20-30 minute Lactic Acid Sessions

Add 1 - 2 x 10– 20 minute ATP-PC Sessions

Here you want to flat out sprint for as long as you can and hold it (between 10 and 20 sec) keeping good form.

You will need 2-3 minutes of recovery between bursts.

I recommend running on flat or hills or spin bike.

Keep up your power and strength training

Add 1-2 x 5-10 min plyometric sessions using exercises that complement your style.

For kicking styles I recommend box jumps, jump squats, touch jumps and tuck jumps.

2- 4 Classes or Skill Specific Training Sessions

4: REST WEEKS

Your body simply cannot go hard all the time as I have talked about in earlier chapters.

It is impossible to maintain peak performance all year round and really you shouldn't want to.

Nobody likes to lose fitness or sharpness, but your body needs recovery time and if you take rest when you need it, you will catch it before injury occurs.

Besides that it can be fun to observe your fitness levels coming back up and each time you do this you learn something new to help you for next time.

Most people can go safely from Phase 1 to 2 without a rest week (although you might need it for a mental holiday), but it is a good idea to take a rest week coming from Phase 2 to 3.

You will not lose any fitness in one week and your body will be better for it.

I'm not a big fan of complete rest for the whole week, so I'd be keeping the slow steady runs, throw in some swims and some walks, you can even drop your weights way back and do some higher reps.

Once you are rested I promise you will be raring and ready to go, both physically and mentally, and enjoy the process a whole lot more.

For workout programs head to **bulletproofconfidencekickassbody.com**

EATING YOUR WAY TO A KICKASS BODY

When I was a Taekwondo competitor my weight division was 43kg – 47kg.

I sat somewhere around the top of that at 46ish on comp day and sat comfortably around 47-48kg the rest of the time.

I'm 165(and a half!!)cm tall and a light frame.

When I began training in Taekwondo I weighed 59kg (ironically the same weight I was the day I gave birth to my son) and while that was still considered thin, I was soft and unfit.

Over the years I had fluctuated between being lean and I guess what you would call 'average'. I have great genes from the maternal side of my family so I was probably able to get away with what most women couldn't and still managed to look okay even if I didn't feel it.

I can remember being on the scales at the gym at around the age of 20 and being told I weighed 46kg; I had been exercising consistently for many months and felt good, but this number meant nothing to me really. I asked the lady, "Is that light?" and she said – well I'm paraphrasing but "der!!"

I fought my first competition roughly six months after starting my training.

I can't remember exactly what weight division I fought under in my first competition, but I think it was roughly under 53kg. I hadn't consciously been trying to lose weight in this time, but it was happening anyway.

At the time I was working a lot of shifts at a local pub and eating and drinking like a person who worked at a pub, but already I was leaner from the training alone.

The closer I got to my black belt, the more seriously I began to take things, the training increased and when it was time to look at black belt weight divisions around 18 months later, I was already sitting pretty close to fly weight – I think I was at 50kg or thereabouts and I knew that with some more attention to my nutrition the last 3kg would come off easily enough.

What I learned from this and even more so later on when I still competed at the same weight after the birth of my kids, (5 months after Cody and 8 months after Chloe), was the balance between needing to drop weight while still maintaining the energy I needed to get quality training sessions in (and be a mum). Without quality training sessions where you feel good, feel strong, feel fit and switched on, things go badly. Remember that competition training is all about full contact sparring, so when you don't have energy or mental sharpness, it is a very bad day at the office and too many of these days can affect your confidence immensely. When you start to string too many of these days together it's all over mentally. Something you want to avoid at all costs because it is very hard to get back.

In your own life away from competition this would translate into no energy to take care of things in your daily life, plus train well and recover well; that feeling of dragging yourself through the day wishing it would end and wondering how the hell you were going to do it all again the next day.

Just cutting calories didn't work for me and more often than not I would eat the same way I normally ate but put in extra training sessions to drop the weight. Back in the day that worked well for me but of course everyone is different, and as I become older this doesn't come as easily to me.

I was lucky enough not to have to go to the lengths some of the other athletes had to go to, to make competition weight. It was not unusual to see athletes running around the streets in garbage bags attempting to sweat off excess weight prior to weigh in. Even after vomiting and dehydration they might still be 100g over.

It was also not unusual to see these competitors in the sauna for hours on end before weigh in. I do not know how some of these athletes even got on the mats some days. Oftentimes they won their fights and hats off to them for being able to tough it out under such tough circumstances, but it wasn't for me that's for sure.

The toughest it got for me was not having brekkie the day of weigh in so I would weigh under 47kg comfortably, although I do remember my instructor/husband eating ice-cream in bed one night and me cracking it at him. My weight must have been a little close for comfort that time around ☺

What I worked out without being too conscious of it, was that good fuel equals good performance and even more so (and highly likely the way I discovered this) the opposite of that, which is bad or lack of fuel equals crap performance, which then leads to a confidence problem we want to avoid.

If you don't currently practice martial arts, for you this could be a bad run, bike ride, swim or crossfit session.

I worked out fast that I was not willing to starve to make weight and any attempt to do so had a major impact on my ability to fight well in training. This led directly to a drop in confidence, something I wanted to avoid at all costs, because training was hard enough without adding that particular brand of mental torture to the mix.

All of this simply from what I did or did not put in my stomach!

It quickly became clear what worked for me and I used this process time and time again. This included LOTS of steamed rice (basmati), grilled chicken breast and broccoli. I reckon I ate that four times a day and never got sick of it and in fact if you were to look in my fridge today you would see five pre-packed serves of exactly that!

I started competing back in the early 90s and since then boy have things come a long way in the world of nutrition and supplementation!

I can remember being at State team training, these were tough 2-hour sessions with lots of sparring, and the thing I can remember about those sessions the most was being soooo thirsty. The Korean instructors didn't want us drinking water (which is what we drank back then) to toughen us up, but looking back now the impact on performance was insane.

These days I still consider an electrolyte drink during training both a luxury and a modern-day miracle and in longer, tougher sessions I wouldn't be without one with added BCAAs (Branch Chain Amino Acids) along with recovery supplements like protein powder and glutamine.

I don't use a ton of supplements, but there are some I don't go without because they work and I'll get to those soon.

No doubt you have heard things like "You can't out train a poor diet" or "Abs are made in the kitchen" or "Abs are 80% diet."

I have to say I don't 100% agree with any of those statements.

I do agree nutrition is crucial and you cannot get the results you want without paying attention to your nutrition, but it is my strong belief that for most people training should be your biggest focus and it is far more important than taking a microscopic approach to your nutrition.

Why?

If you make training and your training goals your number one priority then it becomes all about performance, and good performance is fuelled by good nutrition.

It doesn't matter if your training goal is a fight or a 5km fun run, the same principles still apply.

Even though fun runs aren't entered under a specific weight division, it still makes sense to be at your ideal weight for your best personal performance, doesn't it?

If you want to run 5kms faster than before and without feeling like you are going to die in the process, then it makes sense to be lighter (if you can be) because this puts less stress on your body so you don't have to work as hard.

Getting into the habit of making daily decisions about fuelling your performance by avoiding certain foods and in time heading straight for the foods you know work for you, will all lead to you shedding the weight you want to lose without it all being about counting calories and stepping onto the scales five times a day.

Training the house down and fuelling for performance is a far more empowering and inspiring way to lose weight than the usual methods of starvation, shakes, scale obsession and anything in between of a similar ilk. I urge you to get into this more positive approach mindset, pronto.

If you are not 100% convinced that what you eat dramatically effects your performance (or energy levels) let me suggest a little experiment.

Go a week training at least 90 minutes each day at intensity (can be broken into two sessions) and eat crap or cut out carbs or cut a bunch of calories and see how you get on.

You can do that or you can just take my word for it ☺

Here is what I want for you…

I want you to fall in love with training so hard you are fighting nausea most of the training session (trust me it happens).

I never, ever want you to utter the words "I can't or don't want to go out because I'm on a diet" ever again!

I want you to drop counting calories and avoiding whole food groups and living on meal replacements.

As a bigger picture I want you to think ahead to Christmas time, a time when most people freak out about putting on (more) weight and have a love/hate relationship with the whole festive season, because they fear they have no will power and this will 'undo' all of their hard work.

Hard work that lands them at average usually.

Come Christmas time I want you to imagine looking fit and toned and vibrant and healthy and being able to wear whatever the hell you want, because everything you try on looks amazing.

Now imagine Christmas Day and being able to relax and enjoy eating whatever you want – you have already been for a run or hit the gym or spent time on the bag and you know you will again tomorrow so you have no fear of enjoying a festive meal and wine (if you choose) with your loved ones.

Now imagine New Year's Eve day and you are thinking about the year ahead. Imagine NOT having to set a weight loss goal. I know – crazy isn't it?

Imagine you don't need to set a weight loss goal because you already look and feel smoking hot.

That my friend is where you are headed.

FOOD AS FUEL

The biggest take away I want you to get from all of the above is that training needs to be your priority.

I want you to focus on your performance and recovery without making any big changes to your nutrition for a little while.

Then I want you to start to add in some stuff that will improve performance and recovery.

NOTE: some of you may already have this stuff nailed and reading this next bit may just be confirmation you are on the right track (according to me anyway).

PRE-WORKOUT

When we hit our training session we want to be fuelled up and ready go to (much like a racing car).

We want to be hydrated and have a good supply of glycogen in our muscles, so we have some energy readily available to burn and this is as simple as ensuring you have enough water along with some electrolyte drink, if you think you need it, along with some fast burning carbs and a small amount of protein.

Rye wrap with banana, peanut butter and honey is a popular choice because you are getting fast acting carbs along with some protein.

There will be some instances where you might want to get up and hit your cardio right away on an empty stomach and for some people this works well.

I found through trial and error I ran better with some food in my belly, so have a play around with this yourself to see what works best for you.

INTRA-WORKOUT

During your training session we want to avoid eating into our muscle for energy so taking a BCAA along with an electrolyte drink will do just that. This way you remain hydrated and are protecting precious muscle.

POST-WORKOUT

As I mentioned in the training chapter, when we work at intensity or lift weights we are damaging muscle fibres (that then repair themselves and gain strength) and to help these repair well (this is all about your recovery) we need protein.

I also include the amino acid 'l-glutamine' to help with recovery. The added bonus is it helps support the immune system which can be taxed when we train hard often.

SUPPLEMENTS

Everyone is made differently; your nutrition, the type and frequency of your training, your age and other lifestyle factors will all influence what your specific body needs.

Below are the supplements I take without fail as a base. Rather than notice these supplements doing amazing things, I notice them more when I don't take them.

Electrolyte drinks for hydration.

Multi-Vitamins as a safety net for any gaps in your nutrition.

BCAAs to preserve muscle while training

Protein Powder to help recovery post training.

L-Glutamine to aid in recovery and boost immune system.

Good oils: fish, coconut, flax. These help boost your metabolism.

Below are some other supplements I find useful from time to time:

If I want to gain some muscle I add creatine.

If I'm feeling stressed I add B-Complex.

If I am not getting enough greens in my food I add a green superfood powder to my shakes.

AROUND MEALS

Around meals you want to eat foods that keep your metabolism ticking over and keep you feeling satisfied without feeling heavy.

Here is where you want to address getting enough fruit, veggies and good carbs into your body.

If you are hungry and you can feel your metabolism firing then be sure to add more snacks that are a balance of carbs and protein.

It can be challenging to come up with good snack ideas so I've created a list of 20 of these at the end of the chapter.

PULLING IT ALL TOGETHER
A DAY OF FOOD

PLAN 1

MEAL 1: 1 whole egg

      3 egg whites

      2 cups veggies (spinach, mushroom, tomato – your choice)

      1 slice sprouted grain bread spread with avocado.

      Multi-vitamin/fish oil

MEAL 2: 3 brown rice cakes (thin ones)

      Small can of tuna in olive oil (drained well)

MEAL 3: ½ cup rice

      150g grilled chicken breast

      1 cup of broccoli

      fish oil

MEAL 4: ½ cup mixed berries

      2 tbsp Greek yoghurt

      cinnamon

      dash of organic maple syrup

MEAL 5: 150g steak, fish or chicken breast

      Large salad dressed with balsamic vinegar

      ¼ cup rice (don't have rice on non-training days)

MEAL 6: Protein shake in water with glutamine before bed

PLAN 2

Pre-Training Snack

1 slice toast

1 tsp jam

½ banana

1 tbsp peanut butter

1 tsp coconut oil

AM Workout

Electrolyte drink (can be coconut water) with added BCAAs

Protein and L-Glutamine in water

Breakfast

½ cup oats

115ml milk

½ banana

1 tbsp coconut oil

Protein powder in water

Midmorning Snack

Small handful almonds

1 apple

Lunch

Grain wrap with chicken breast and salad

Late Afternoon Snack

½ cup cottage cheese

½ banana

¼ cup Greek yoghurt

honey

PM Workout

Electrolyte drink (can be coconut water)

With added BCAAs.

Protein and L-Glutamine in water

Dinner

Salad or steamed veggies and lean protein plus ¼ cup brown rice

Evening Snack

¾ cup cottage cheese

1 cup mixed berries

WORKOUT SUPPLEMENTATION

If I train once a day then I only supplement once.

If I train twice I supplement twice.

NOTE: You can avoid protein shakes altogether if you wish and simply use protein based foods instead. I like the convenience of protein powders and they work well for me, but you need to determine for yourself if this is for you or not.

This might seem like an awful lot of food to some women, but remember we are training HARD and often.

Two workouts a day most days and we constantly need to refuel for both performance and recovery.

Ladies, here is where SIZE DOES MATTER!

This amount of food and these serving sizes work for me because my metabolism is fast (I had this tested and my metabolism is quite high) and on top of my training sessions each day I'm hard put to sit still for 20 minutes at a time, so I'm always up and down and running around and this burns calories too.

If your metabolism is slower, you are training less or are sedentary most of the day, then you may not get away with eating these portion sizes and you may need to drop your serving sizes back.

If you only workout out once a day then drop the second workout nutrition.

DON'T skip meals or drop snacks, instead adjust the size.

We want to keep our energy levels consistent throughout the day with light and healthy meals and snacks, dump some good fast-burning carbs into our bodies before training times to fuel for the workout and then dump in some protein afterwards to fuel for recovery.

It really is as simple as that, so don't make it more complicated than it needs to be.

It can be daunting for those of you who have obsessively avoided carbs or have been living on reduced calories and have counted every calorie that passes your lips (all the while starving yourself to death), but I want to ask you…

What have you been doing up to now… how is that working out for you?

If what you are doing works for you then stick with it, but if not, it's time to try something different… so why not this?

If you have royally screwed your metabolism from under eating or avoiding any form of carbohydrate, then you may have an initial increase in weight as your metabolism takes time to catch up. You will need to make sure your portion sizes are appropriate and hang in there, it will turn around.

Unfortunately messing up and then righting a banged-up metabolism can be like turning around a ship going along at full speed; it's hard to pull up and even harder to get going again.

While it looks like nothing much is happening and that things aren't moving, below deck the engine is cranking and doing its darndest to get the thing moving again, and over time the boat once again picks up speed and motors along as it should.

When you feel nothing is happening, just hang in there and tough it out.

If we continue to use the ship analogy can you imagine what would happen if the captain cut the engine time and time again because he didn't think he was getting anywhere?

The ship would come to a complete standstill until the captain started her up again and then he would cut the engine again as soon as he thinks there is no progress being made.

What do you suppose happens when this happens? He gets nowhere fast is what happens.

If he hadn't stuffed about stopping and starting the captain would have seen the boat was in fact moving and slowly gaining speed every step of the way.

Had he just kept moving forwards instead of stopping and starting he would have been well on his way much sooner.

It is exactly the same thing with your metabolism. Stick at it and don't stop and start because every time you do you mess with any progress you have been making, whether or not you could see it.

My last word on nutrition is this…

Everybody wants a quick-fix, lose-weight-fast-and-keep-it-off-forever answer, but there simply isn't one. Good nutrition takes time and effort and trial and error. There are no shortcuts, but once you get this worked out there is also no looking back.

What I have offered above has worked for me and for others time and time again, but you will only arrive at what works best for you by following the guidelines I have listed above and tweaking them to suit you.

Don't become disheartened or give up when the going gets tough.

When overwhelm kicks in go right back to basics and follow one of the pre-set meal plans included in the book. Once you get back on top of things you can start to experiment again. Really what you are looking for is what foods leave you feeling great and what foods leave you feeling bloated, overfull and heavy. Eat more of the foods that leave you feeling good and none of the foods that don't.

Give yourself months rather than days or weeks to get it right. You will still make progress in that time but fully understanding what works for your body to support you during training and recovery often takes a while. Sometimes we miss the feedback our body is giving us in the early days and it can take until our nutrition is much cleaner before we notice, so hang in there. I promise the time and effort will be worth it.

20 PROTEIN/CARB BALANCED SNACKS

1: ½ cup cottage cheese and ½ cup mixed berries or banana

2: 2 egg whites and an apple

3: Tuna in springwater on 1 slice grain toast

4: Babybel cheese (kids size) and an apple

5: Low fat cheese slice on 4 grain crackers

6: ½ cup Greek yoghurt with drizzle of honey and a banana

7: 1 whole egg and a large carrot

8: Protein powder in skim milk

9: Protein powder in water and 6 dried apricots

10: 10 almonds and a pear

11: 1 tbsp natural peanut butter and an apple

12: 1 cup of strawberries and ½ cup Greek yoghurt

13: 2 rice cakes with 1 tbsp natural peanut butter

14: Grain English muffin with peanut butter

15: Grain English muffin with grilled light cheese

16: Protein pancake made with oats (from recipes)

17: Protein Ball and an apple (from recipes)

18: 2 Vitawheat biscuits with ½ cup cottage cheese

19: 50g chicken breast and ½ grapefruit

20: 1 glass of skim milk and a banana

ABOUT THE AUTHOR

5th Degree Black Belt, Michelle Hext, grew up amidst domestic violence, sexual abuse and poverty. She left school at 14 years of age and home at the age of 16.

Since then she has worked hard to live a meaningful and inspirational life.

Going back to school, learning to fly an aeroplane and traveling overseas alone all came before beginning her beloved Taekwondo in 1991.

Since then her life has been dedicated to practicing Taekwondo, its principles and the lessons it has taught her along with way.

Michelle has been practicing Taekwondo for 22 years as student, sparring competitor and instructor; she is ranked 5th Degree Black Belt in WTF Taekwondo.

Michelle has been a personal trainer for over 18 years and was one of Australia's first online personal trainers; she is also a trained life coach.

Today Michelle is the founder of the only female-only dojang in Australia (PUSH Women's Only Taekwondo). She is also founder and editor of Black Belt Woman Mag, a digital magazine for women in Martial Arts.

Michelle is a 44-year-old mother of two teenagers, Cody 17 and Chloe 15.

For more information please visit **www.MichelleHext.com** and **BulletproofConfidenceKickassBody.com**

www.ingramcontent.com/pod-product-compliance
Lightning Source LLC
Chambersburg PA
CBHW060910280326
41934CB00007B/1261